Acupuncture

MERIDIANS and POINTS

经络腧穴

Sumiko Knudsen

Ph.D
Practitioner, DK

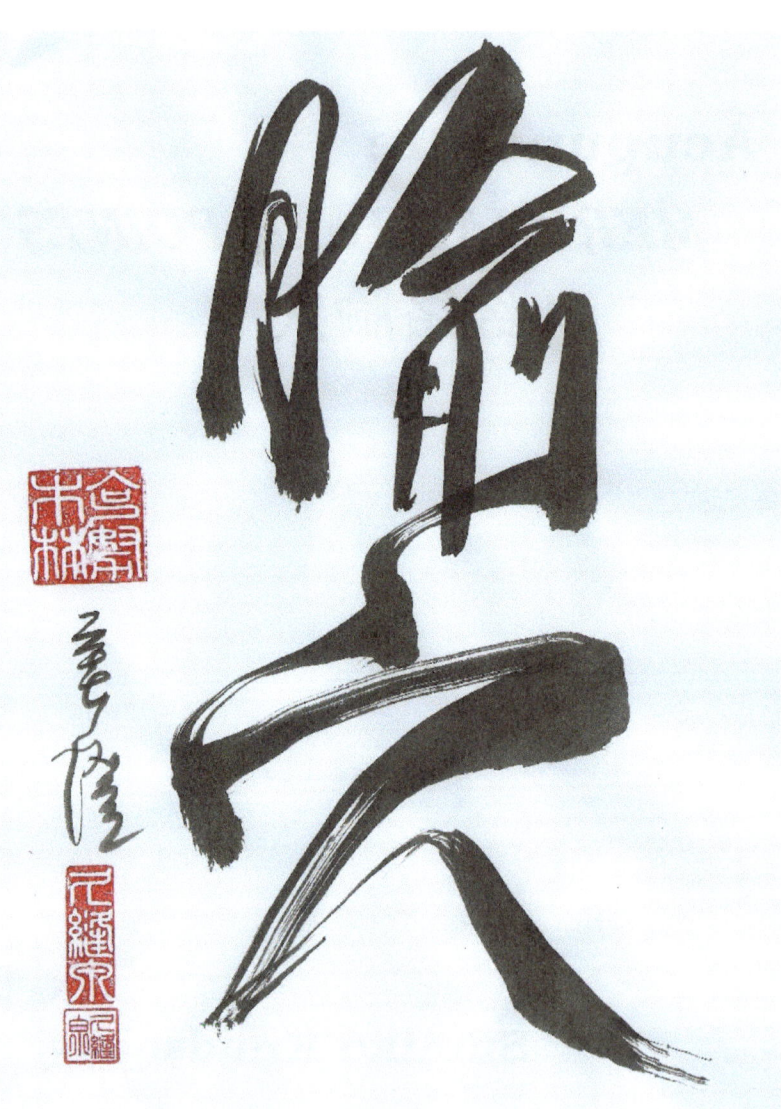

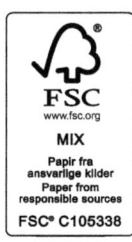

2019 © Sumiko Knudsen
Publisher: BoD – Copenhagen, Denmark
Printing: BoD – Norderstedt, Germany

ISBN: 9788743012016

CONTENTS

INTRODUCTION

Acupuncture points are the places where acupuncture needle is applied for the treatment of diseases. This acupuncture point location and the therapeutic result are related.

Acupuncture point locations are related to Qi and Blood flowing and this energy system defined pathway from internal organs and meridians converges and disperses.

Therefore, the locations of acupuncture points are certainly related to physiological functions. Stimulating acupoints in meridians of the affected area may be effective and stimulate meridian points for each disease to approach the affected area.

Stimulation through acupuncture points can correct imbalance and blockages in the flow of energy for restoring health.

WHO in their standard acupuncture nomenclature identifies the 14 main meridians, 361 classical acupuncture points, 48 extra points, 8 extra meridians and Scalp acupuncture lines.

Sumiko Knudsen 克努森澄子

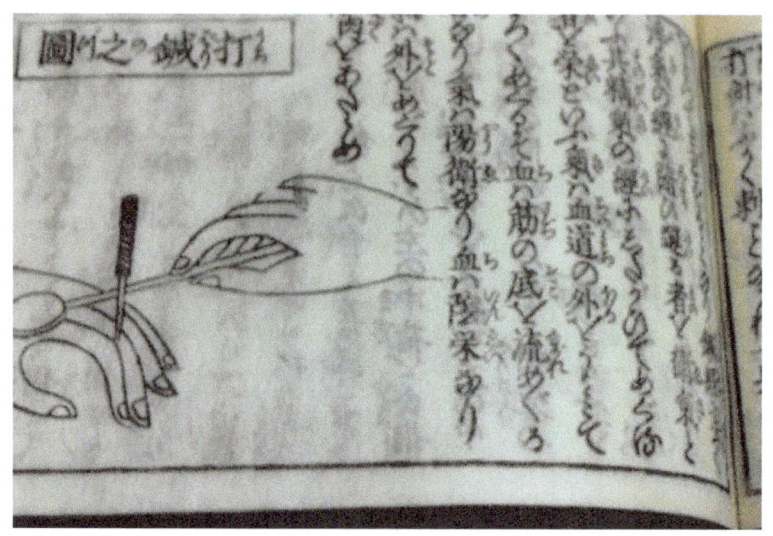

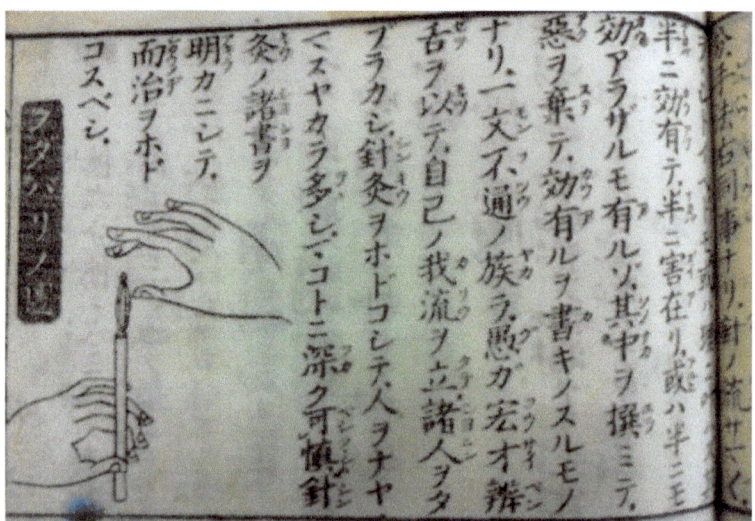

Edo period about 1600

1 Methods of Acupuncture points location 腧穴定位的方法

There are three methods of Acupuncture point location which are used in clinic at present.

1. Anatomical Landmarks 骨度 折量定位法

Anatomical landmarks include 2 landmarks which are Fixed landmarks and Moving landmarks.

1) Fixed landmarks

Fixed landmarks which would not change with body movement. It is five sensory organs, hair, nails, nipple, umbilicus, and prominence and depression of the bones. They are for example, Ex 1 印堂 (Yintang), Du 25 素髎 (Suliao) and Ren 8 神阙 (Shenque)).

2) Moving landmarks

It refers to appear when the part of body keeps in a specific position, and for example, when the arm is flexed and the cubital crease appear, LI-11 曲池 (Quchi). SI-3 后溪 (Houxi) which is made from fist, the point is at the end of the distal transverse crease of the palm.

2. Proportional Measurements 指寸定位法

Human body which is width and length of various portions of the body are divided respectively into definite numbers of proportional measurement. These are standard on any sexes, age and body sizes for patients.

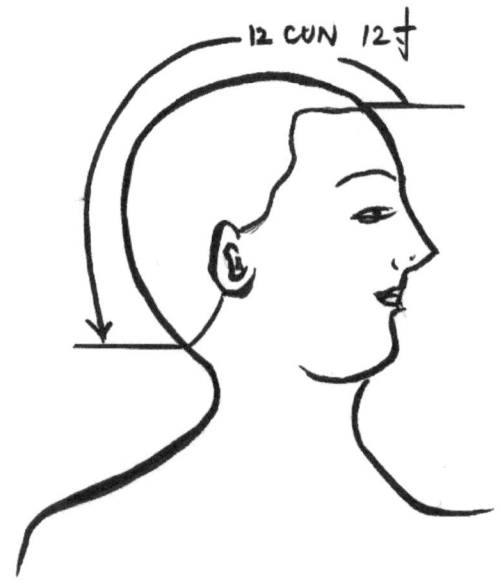

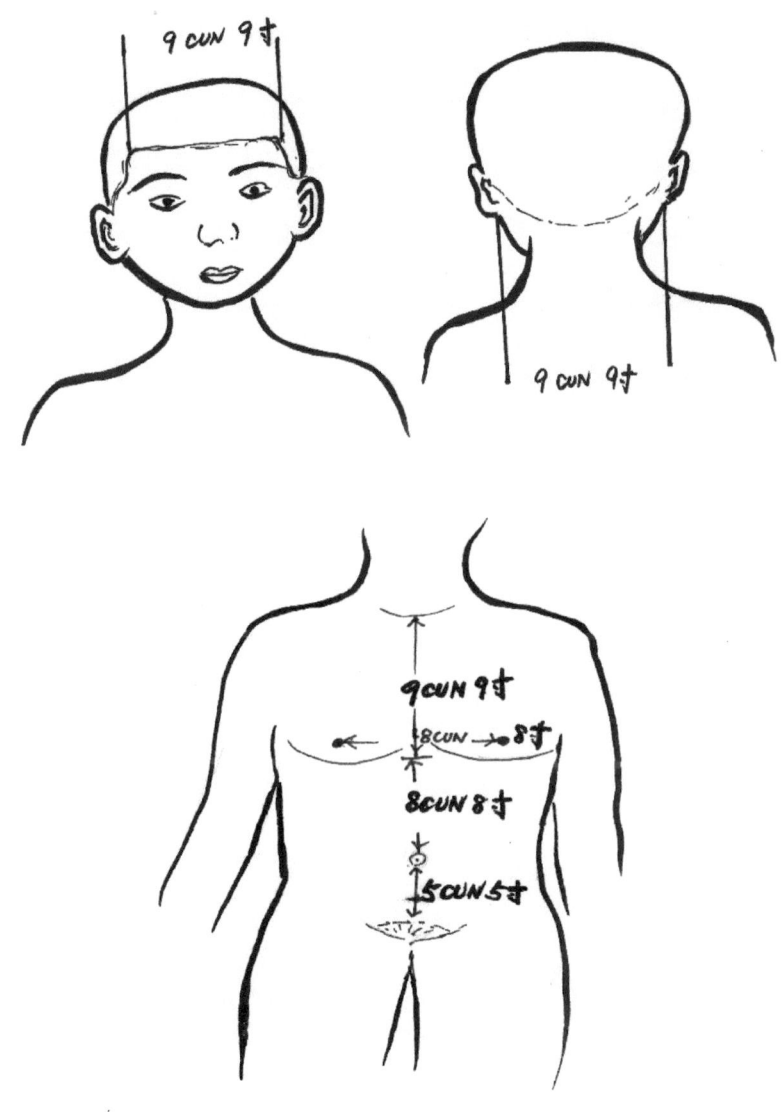

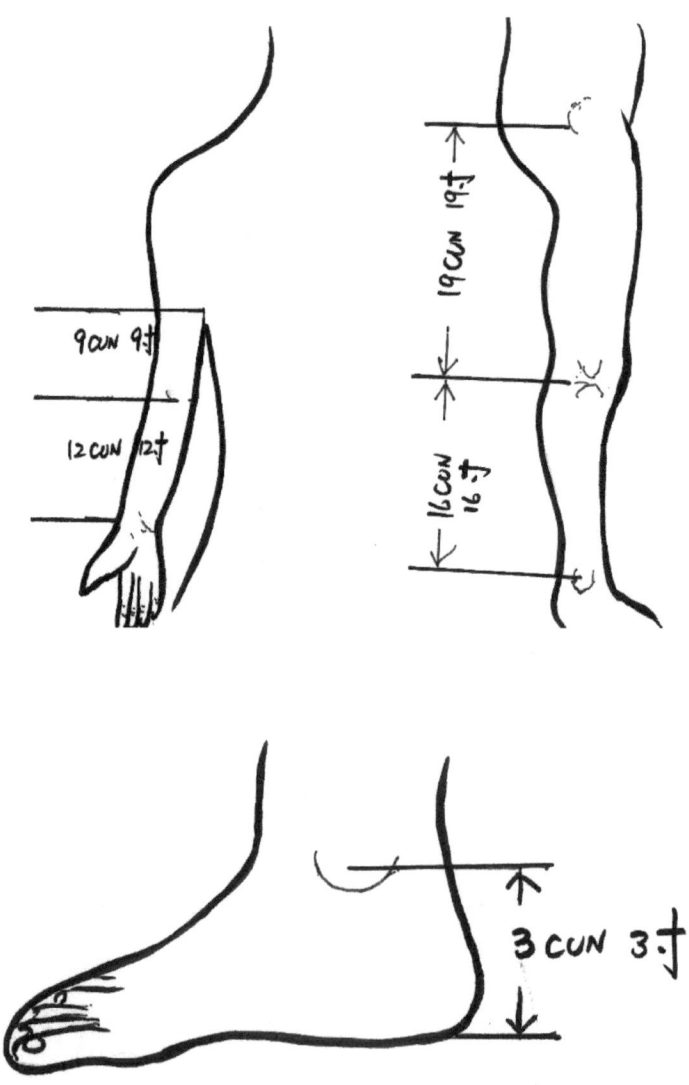

9 CUN 9寸

12 CUN 12寸

19 CUN 19寸

16 CUN 16寸

3 CUN 3寸

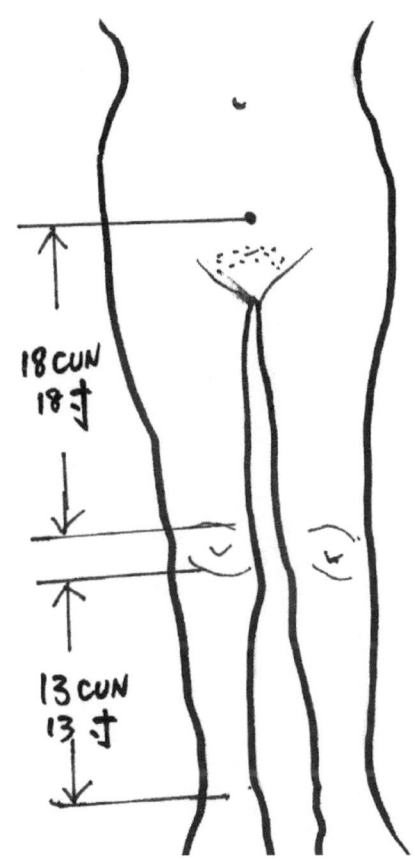

18 CUN
18 寸

13 CUN
13 寸

3. Finger Measurements 指寸定位法

1) Thumb measurement

The width of the thumb is taken as one cun.

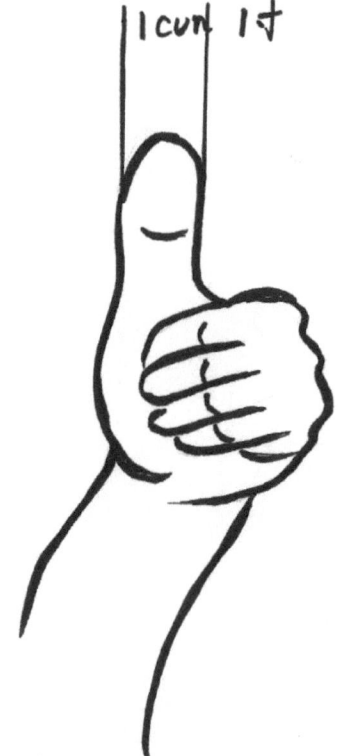

2) Four finger measurement

The width of the four fingers such as index, middle, ring and little are used. Those fingers should be close together to the middle finger and are taken as three cun.

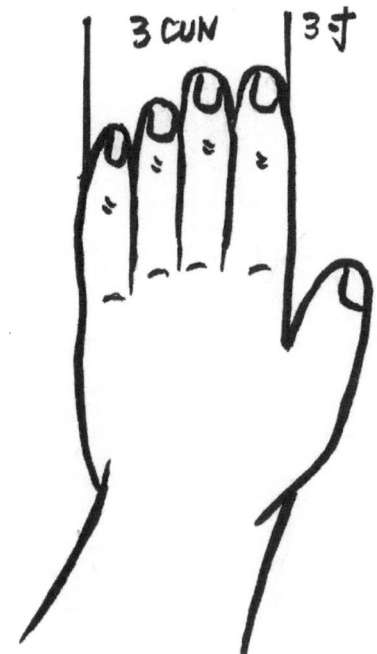

3) Middle finger measurement

The middle finger is flexed, and the distance between two medial ends of the crease of the interphalangeal joint is taken as 1 cun.

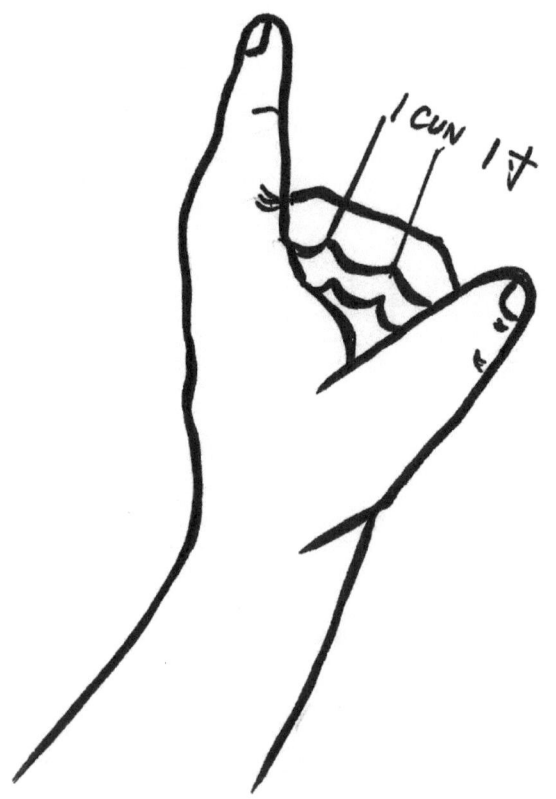

Section 2   Specific Points 特定穴

Specific points refer to fourteen channels which have properties and grouped. They are classified into limbs and head and trunk.

1. Specific points on the Limbs

1.1   Five Shu Points 五输穴

each of the twelve main channels has five Shu points which are Jing-Well, Ying-Spring, Shu-Stream, Jing-River and He-Sea. In addition, there are Lower He-Sea points.

1.2   Yuan-Primary Points 原穴

Each of the twelve main channels has a Yuan-Primary point, and they are taken to treat disorders of the Zang-Fu organs.

1.3   Luo-Connecting Points 络穴

Each of the twelve main channels has a Luo-connecting point, and they are taken to treat disorders of the two exterior-interior related channels.

1.4   Xi-Cleft Points 郄穴

Xi-Cleft points where the Qi and Blood of the channel are deeply converged are used to treat acute disorders.

1.5 Ashi Points 啊是穴

Ashi points are the points of pain. "Where there is a painful spot, there is an acupuncture point" by Yellow emperor.

2. Specific points on the Head and Trunk

2.1 Back-Shu Points 背俞穴

Back-Shu points are specific points on the back where the Qi of the Zang-Fu organs is infused.

2.2 Front-Mu Points 募穴

Front-Mu points are on the chest and abdomen where the Qi of the Zang-Fu organs is infused.

Section 3 Fourteen channels
Location of the Points 十四经穴的定位
I. The Lung Channel of Hand Taiyin
手太阴肺经经穴

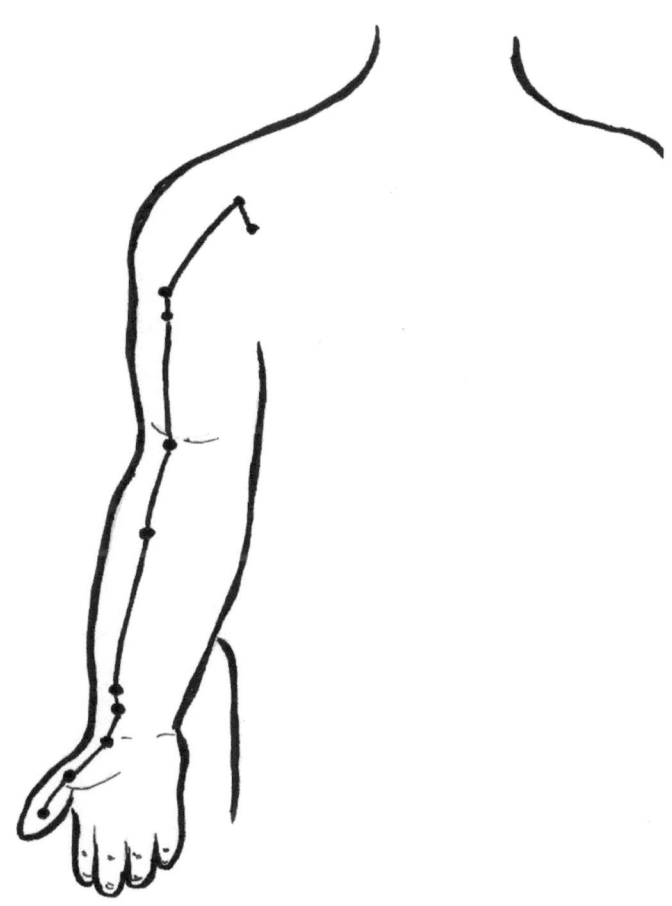

Starts on the chest near the armpit and it goes continuously downward the forearm to end of medial side of the tip of the thumb. It contains 11 different acupoints.

LU-1 (Zhongfu 中府)

- Front-Mu point
- On the lateral aspect of the chest in the first intercostal space, 1 cun directly below LU-2, 6 cun lateral to the anterior midline.

LU-2 (Yunmen 云门)

- On the antero-lateral aspect of the chest, there is a depression the shape of triangle at the lower lateral of the clavicle, 6 cun lateral to the midline.

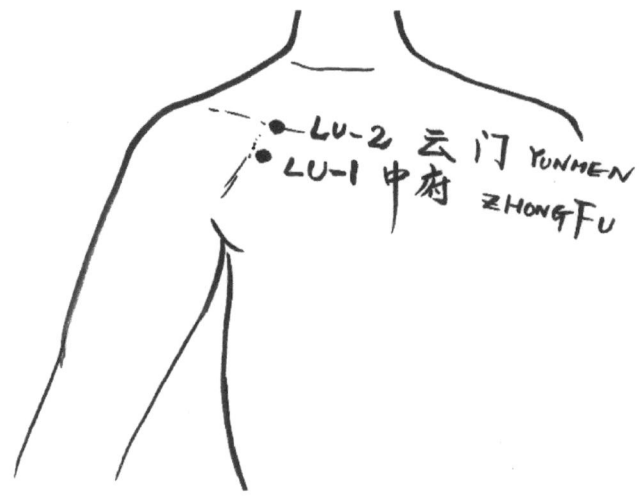

LU-3 (Tianfu 天府)

- On the medial aspect of the upper arm, 3 cun inferior to the end of the axillary fold, radial side of the biceps brachii.

  When raising the arm forward, touch the radial side of the biceps brachii with the tip of the nose.

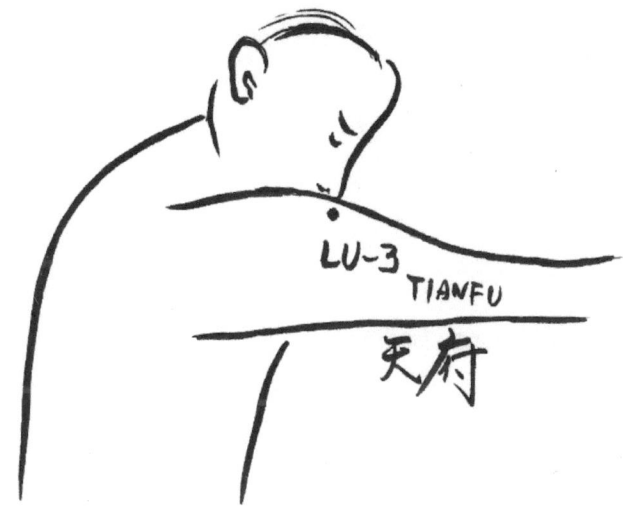

LU-4 (Xiabai 侠白)

- With the upper arm flexed, it is located 1 cun below LU-3.

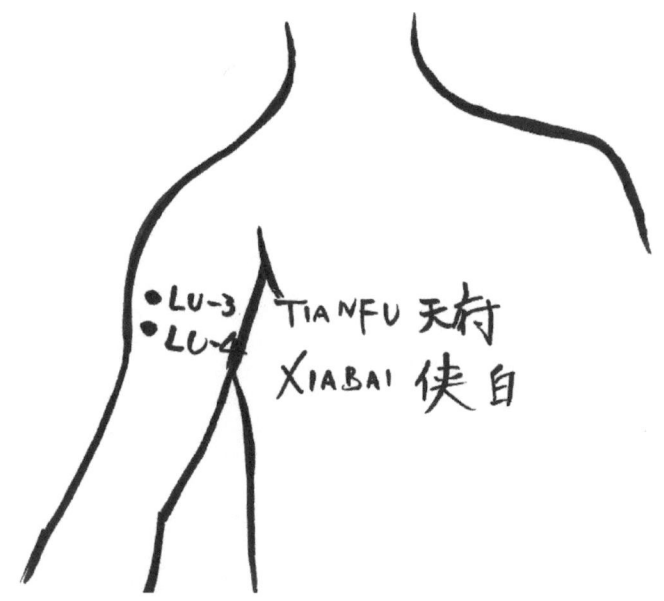

LU-5 (Chize 尺泽)

- He Sea point
- On the transverse cubital crease, in the depression at the radial side of the tendon of biceps brachii.

LU-6 (Kongzui 孔最)

- Xi-Cleft point

- On the medial border of the radius, along the line connection LU-5, 5 cun below. 7 cun above the LU-9.

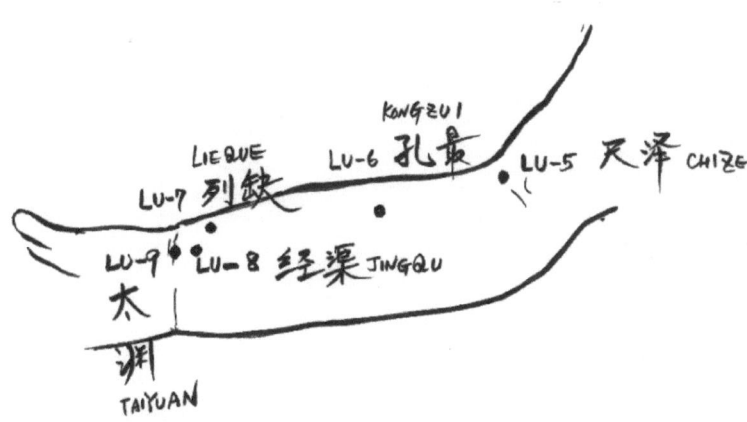

LU-7 (Lieque 列缺)

- Luo-Connecting point
- On the radial aspect of the forearm 1.5 cun above the transverse crease of the wrist between two tendons.

When the index fingers and thumbs of both hands are crossed with the other hand, LU-7 is right under the tip of the index finger.

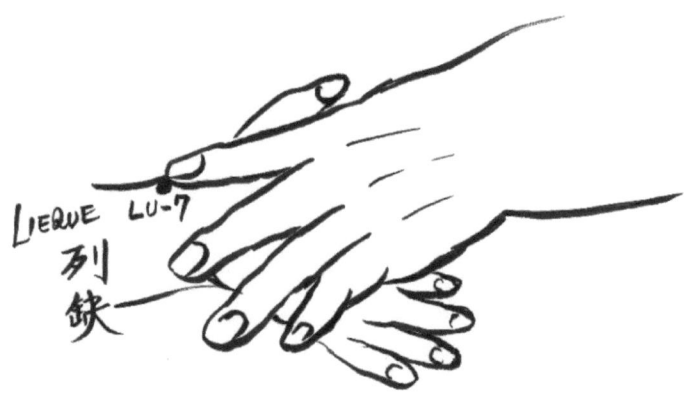

LU-8 (Jingqu 经渠)

- 1 cun above the transverse crease of the wrist, in the depression on the lateral side of the radial artery.

LU-9 (Taiyuan 太渊)

- Yuan-Primary point
- At the radial end of transvers crease of the wrist, in the depression on the radial side of the radial artery.

LU-10 (Yuji 鱼际)

- At the radial aspect of the midpoint of the first metacarpal bone, on the junction of the red and white skin.

LU-11 (Shaoshang 少商)

- On the radial side of the thumb, 0.1 cun from the corner of the nail.

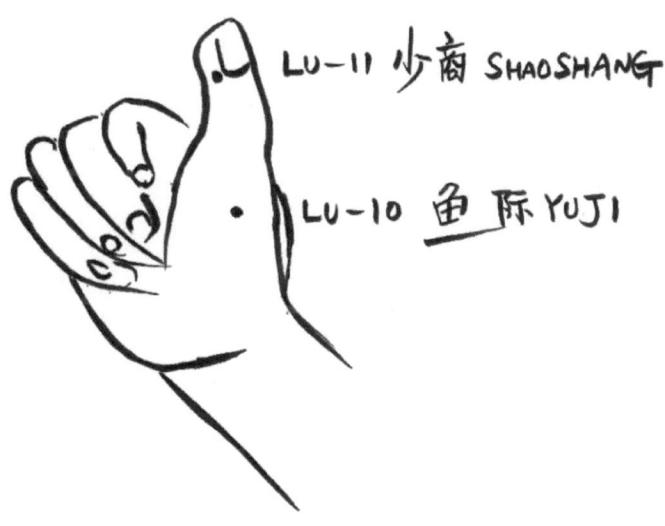

II. The Large Intestine Channel of Hand-Yangming 手阳明大肠经经穴

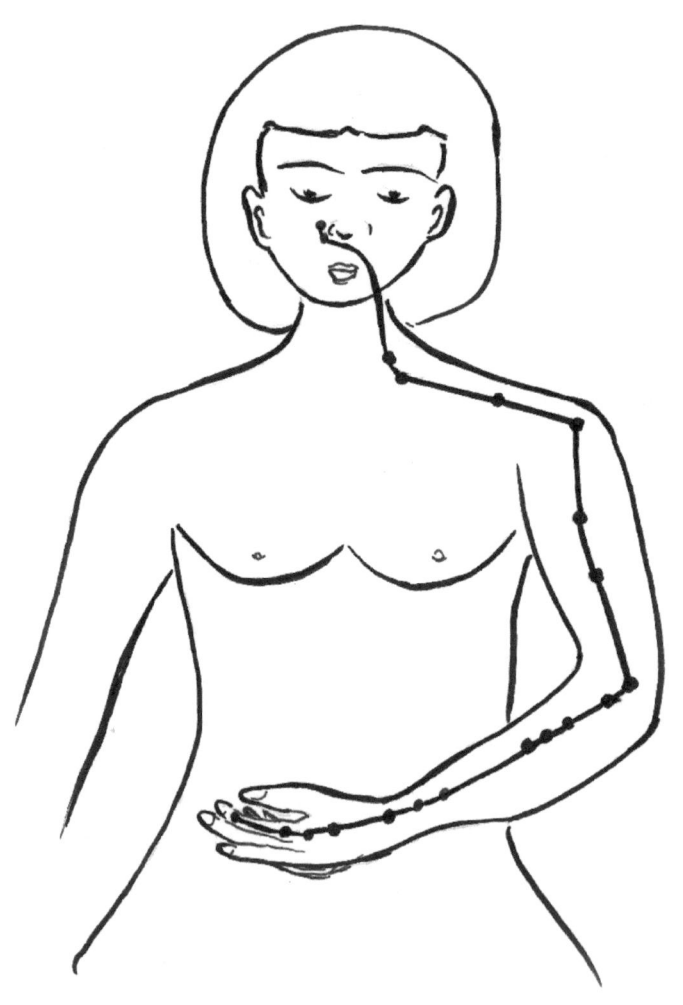

Starts at the tip of the index finger along the upper side of the arm to the highest point of the shoulder, runs upward to the neck, passes through the cheek to the nose. It contains 20 different acupoints.

Li-1 (Shangyang 商阳)

- On the radial side of the index finger, 0.1 cun beside the corner of the nail.

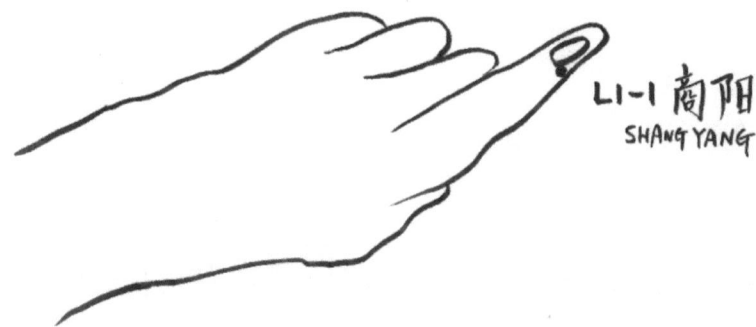

Li-2 (Erjian 二间)

- On the radial side of the index finger, in the depression distal to the second metacarpal-phalangeal joint. Point locates slightly flexed.

Li-3 (Sanjian 三间)

- On the radial side of the index finger, in the depression proximal to the second metacarpal-phalangeal joint.

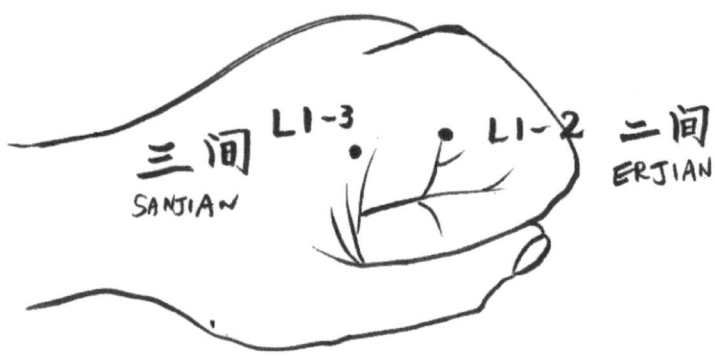

Li-4 (Hegu 合谷)

- Yuan-Primary point.
- On the dorsum of the hand between the first and second metacarpal bones, locate the point to stretch both thumbs and index finger of the left hand, place the transvers crease of the interphalangeal joint of the right thumb

on the margin of the web between the left hand. The point is where the tip of the thumb touches.

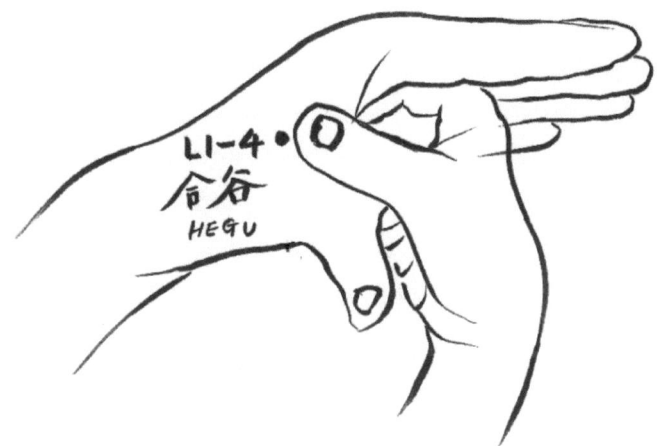

Li-5 (Yangxi 阳溪)

- On the radial side of the wrist, when the thumb is tilted upward, it is the depression between the tendons of extensor pollicis longus and brevis.

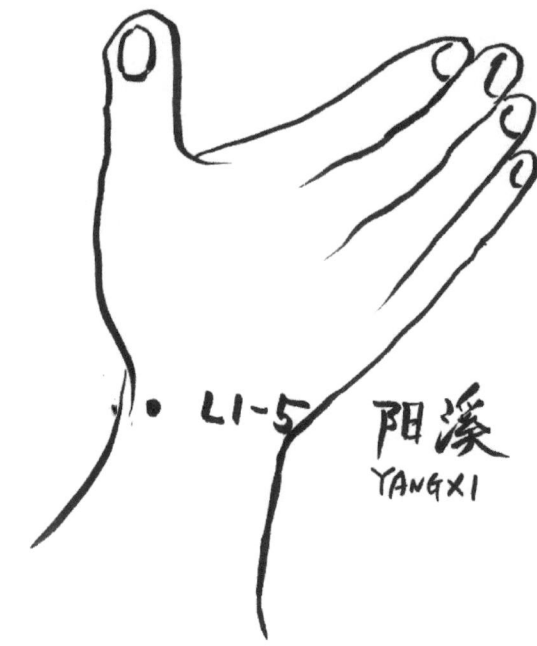

LI-5 阳溪 YANGXI

Li-6 (Pianli 偏历)

- Luo-Connecting point.
- On the radial side of dorsal surface of the forearm, 3 cun proximal to the wrist crease.

Li-7 (Wenliu 温溜)

- Xi-Cleft point.

- On the radial side of dorsal surface of the forearm, 5 cun proximal to the wrist crease.

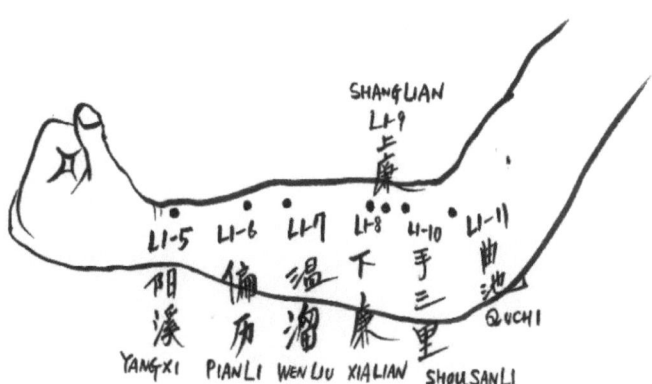

Li-8 (Xialian 下廉)

- On the radial side of dorsal surface of the forearm, 4 cun distal to the cubital crease.

Li-9 (Shanglian 上廉)

- On the radial side of dorsal surface of the forearm, 3 cun distal to the cubital crease.

Li-10 (Shousanli 手三里)

- On the radial side of dorsal surface of the forearm, 2 cun distal to the cubital crease.

Li-11 (Quchi 曲池)

- He-Sea point.
- In the depression at the lateral end of the transverse cubital crease

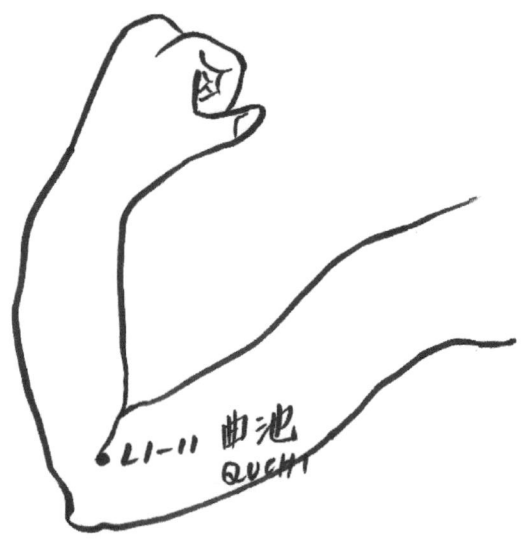

Li-12 (Zhouliao 肘髎)

- On the lateral side of the upperarm, 1 cun above to LI-11(Quchi 曲池).

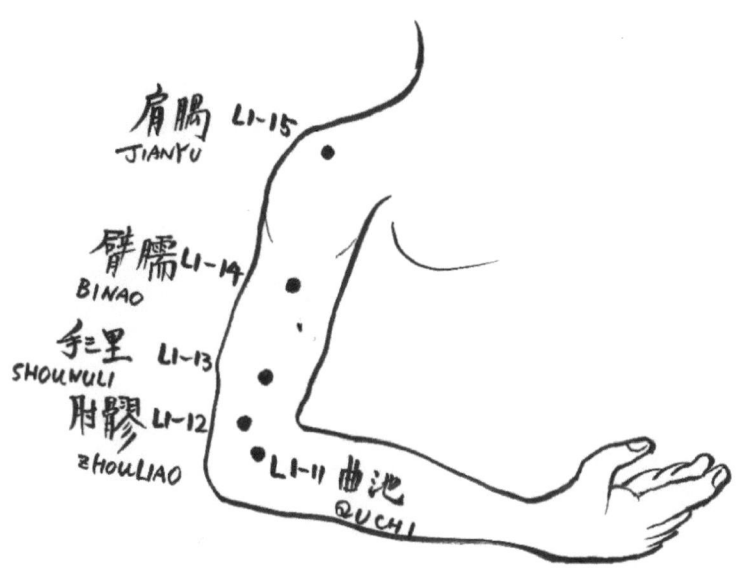

Li-13 (Shouwuli 手五里)

- On the lateral side of the upperarm, 3 cun above to LI-11(Quchi 曲池).

Li-14 (Binao 臂臑)

- On the lateral side of the upperarm, on the line joining LI-11 (Quchi 曲池) and LI-15 (Jianyu 肩髃), 7 cun above LI-11 (Quchi 曲池).

Li-15 (Jianyu 肩髃)

- On the shoulder, in the depression anterior border of the acromioclavicular point.

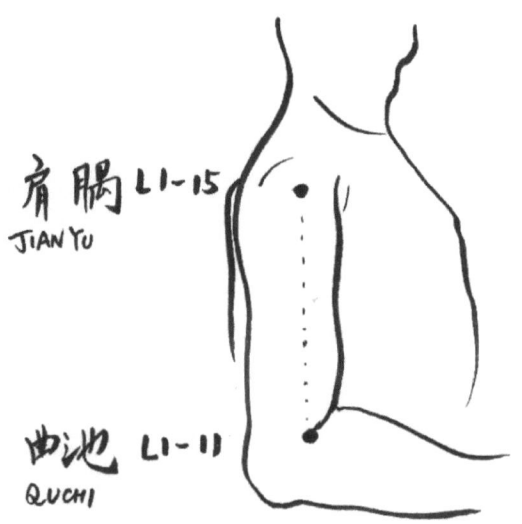

Li-16 (Jugu 巨骨)

- On the shoulder, in the depression between the acromial extremity of the clavicle and the scapular spine

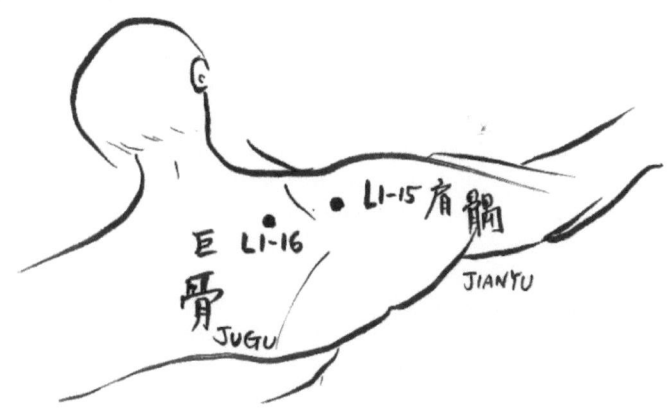

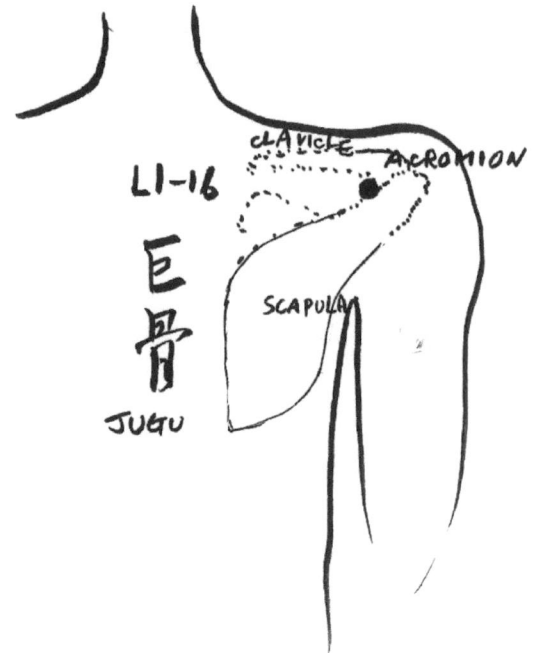

Li-17 (Tianding 天鼎)

- On the lateral side of the neck, at the posterior border of the sternocleidomastoid muscle. 1 cun inferior to Li-18 (Futu 扶突).

Li-18 (Futu 扶突)

- On the lateral side of the neck, level with the tip of Adam's apple between the anterior and posterior borders of the sternocleidomastoid muscle.

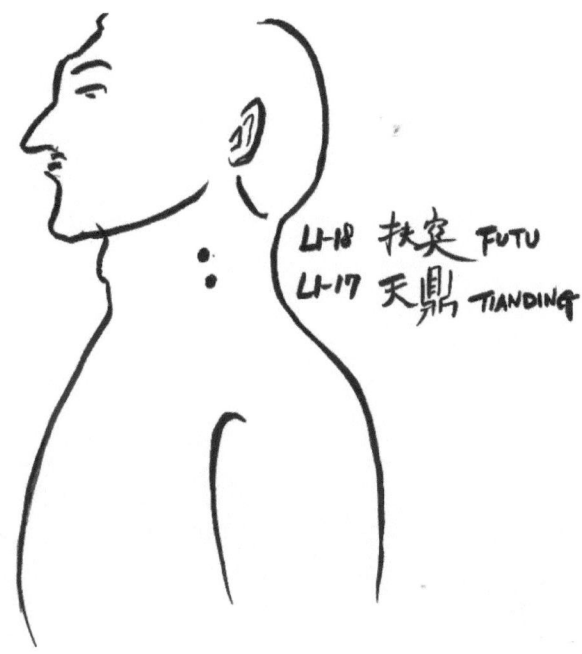

LI-18 扶突 FUTU
LI-17 天鼎 TIANDING

Li-19 (Kouheliao 口禾髎)

- Below the lateral border of the nostril and near the upper lip, at the level of Du-26 (Renzong 人中).

Li-20 (Yingxiang 迎香)

- In the naso-labial groove, at the level of the midpoint of the ala nasi.

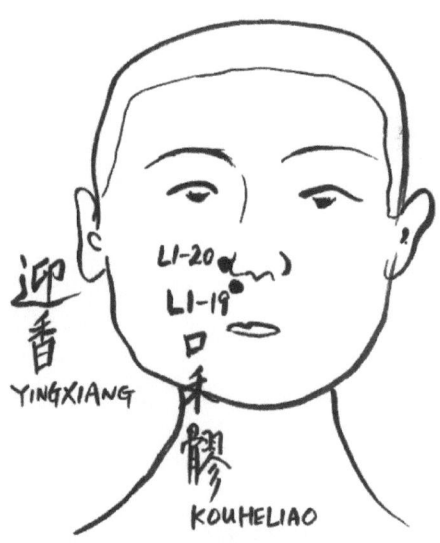

III. The Stomach Channel of Foot-Yangming 足阳明胃经经穴

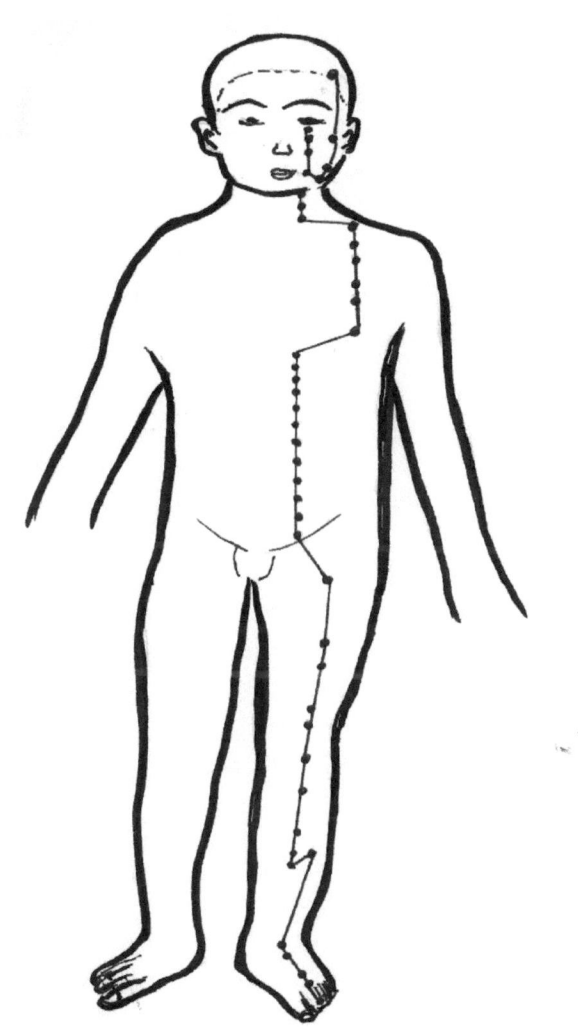

Starts below the pupil of the eye and then to the nose to the jaw, where it splits. The one goes up the scalp but the other one runs down to the neck, chest, abdomen, thigh and through down to the side of the tip of the second toe. It contains 45 different acupoints.

ST-1 (Chengqi 承泣)

- With the eyes looking straight forward, the point is directly   below the pupil between the eyeball and the infraorbital ridge.

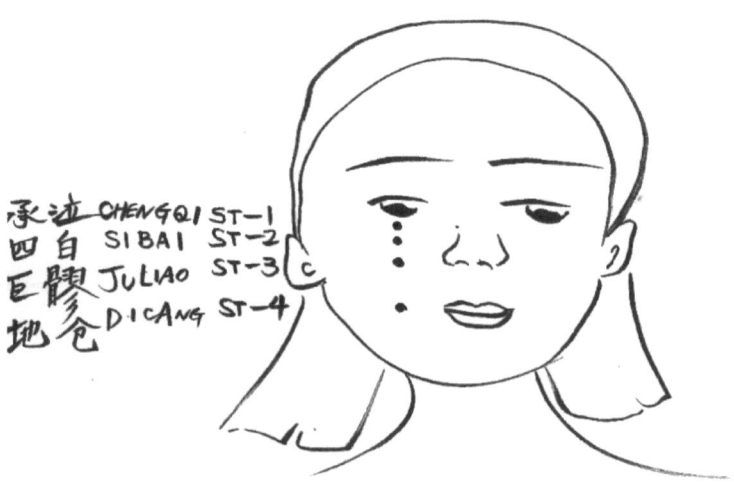

ST-2 (Sibai 四白)

- With the eyes looking straight forward, the point is directly below the pupil, in the depression of the infraorbital foramen.

ST-3 (Juliao 巨髎)

- With the eyes looking straight forward, the point is directly below the pupil, level of the lower border of the ala nasi on the lateral side of the naso-labial groove.

ST-4 (Dicang 地仓)

- Lateral corner of the mouth.

ST-5 (Daying 大迎)

- Anterior to the angle of the mandible, in the depression at the anterior border of the masseter muscle.

ST-6 (Jiache 颊车)

- One finger-breadth anterior and superior to the angle of the mandible.

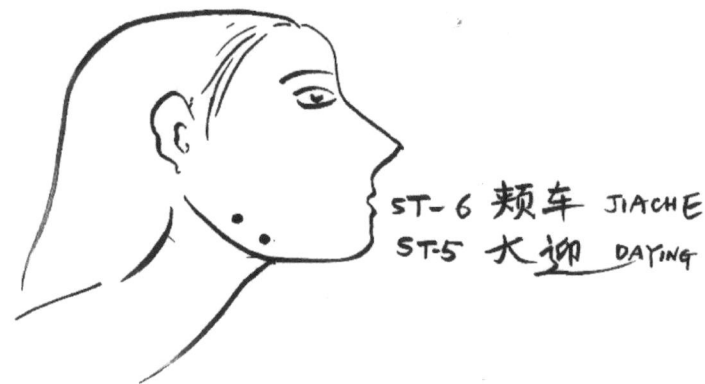

ST-6 颊车 JIACHE
ST-5 大迎 DAYING

ST-7 (Xiaguan 下关)

- Anterior to the ear on the face, in the depression between zygomatic arch and mandibular notch.

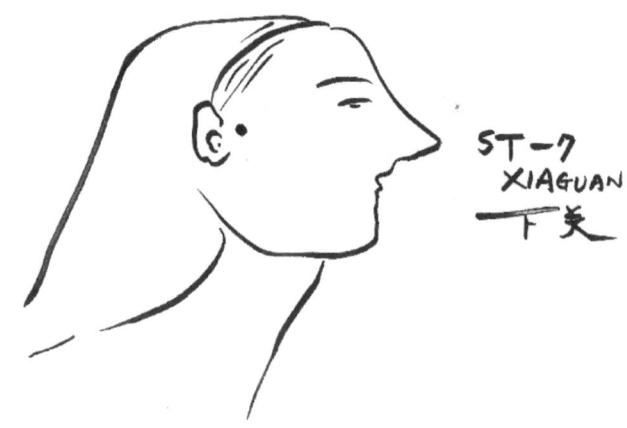

ST-7
XIAGUAN
下关

ST-8 (Touwei 头维)

- 0.5 cun above the anterior hairline at the corner of the forehead.

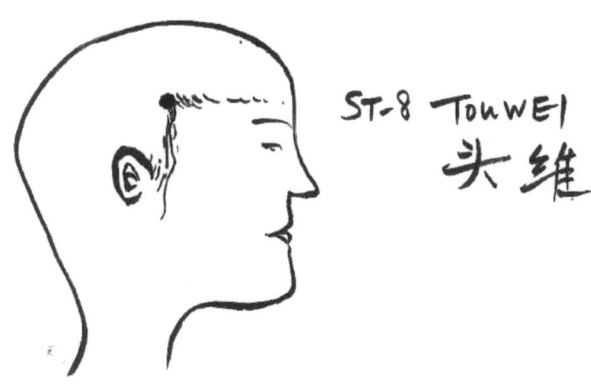

ST-9 (Renying 人迎)

- Level with the tip of Adam apple, on the anterior border of the sternocleidomastoid muscle where the common carotid artery is palpable.

ST-10 (Shuitu 水突)

- On the neck, on the anterior border of the sternocleidomastoid muscle, midpoint of the line ST-9 (Renying 人迎) and ST-11 (Qishe 气舍).

ST-11 (Qishe 气舍)

- On the neck, superior to the medial end of the clavicle, directly under ST-9 (Renying 人迎) between the sternal and clavicular heads of the sternocleidomastoid muscle.

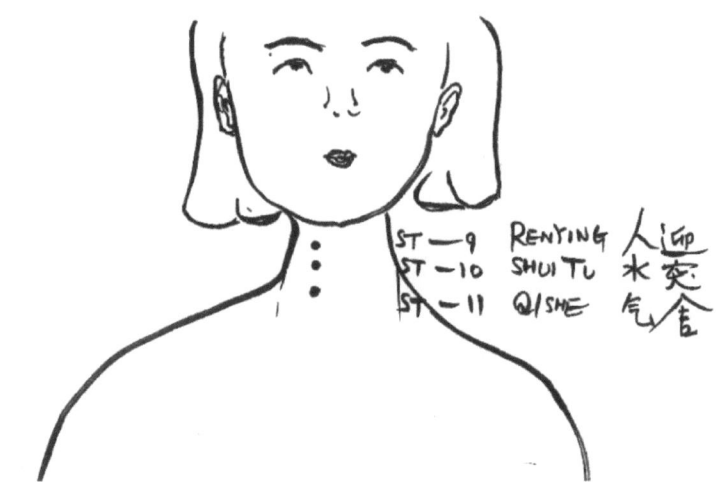

ST-12 (Quepen 缺盆)

- This point is at the midpoint of the supraclavicular fossa, 4 cun lateral to the midline.

ST-13 (Qihu 气户)

- This point is at the midpoint of the lower border of the clavicle, directly below ST-12 (Quepen 缺盆). 4 cun lateral to the midline.

ST-14 (Kufang 库房)

- On the chest, in the first intercostal space, 4 cun lateral to the anterior midline.

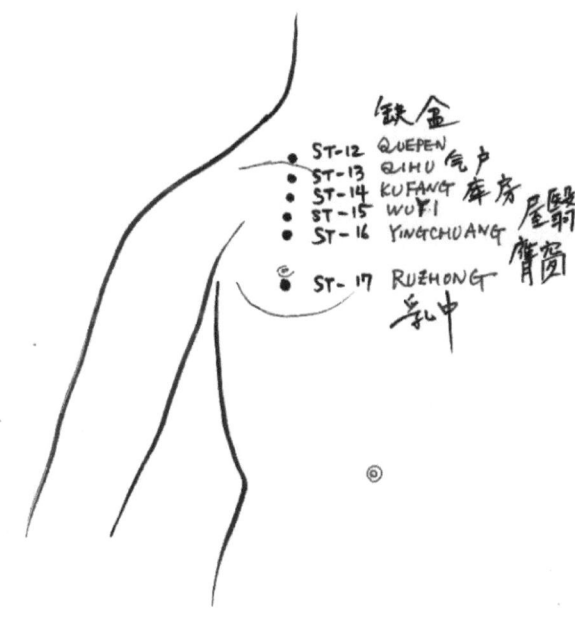

ST-15 (Wuyi 屋翳)

- On the chest, in the second intercostal space, 4 cun lateral to the anterior midline.

ST-16 (Yingchuang 膺窗)

- On the chest, in the third intercostal space, 4 cun lateral to the anterior midline.

ST-17 (Ruxhong 乳中)

- On the chest, in the fourth intercostal space, at the corner of the nipple, 4 cun lateral to the anterior midline.

ST-18 (Rugen 乳根)

- On the chest, directly below the nipple, in the fifth intercostal space.

ST-19 (Burong 不容)

- On the upper abdomen, 6 cun above the umbilicus, 2 cun lateral to the anterior midline.

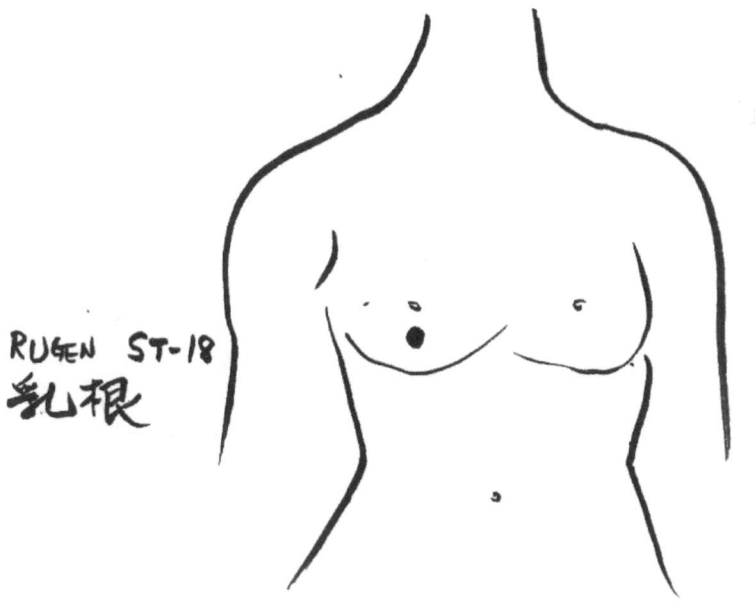

RUGEN ST-18
乳根

ST-20 (Chengman 承满)

- On the upper abdomen, 5 cun above the umbilicus, 2 cun lateral to the anterior midline.

ST-21 (Liangmen 梁门)

- On the abdomen, 4 cun above the umbilicus, 2 cun lateral to the anterior midline.

ST-22 (Guanmen 关门)

- On the abdomen, 3 cun above the umbilicus, 2 cun lateral to the anterior midline.

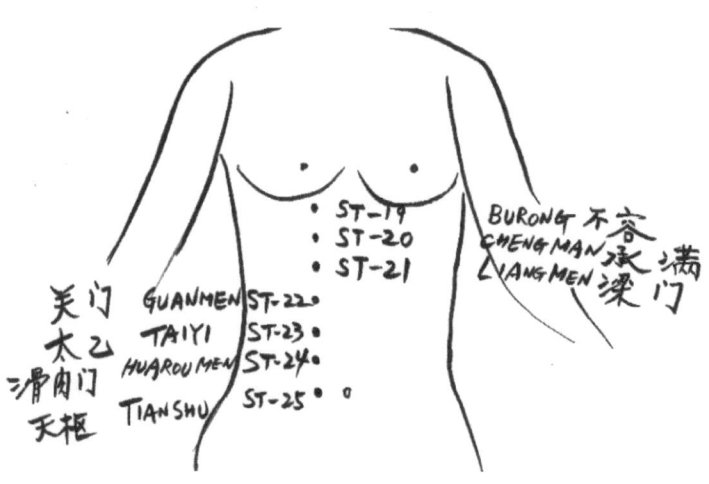

ST-23 (Taiyi 太乙)

- On the abdomen, 2 cun above the umbilicus, 2 cun lateral to the anterior midline.

ST-24 (Huaroumen 滑肉门)

- On the abdomen, 1 cun above the umbilicus, 2 cun lateral to the anterior midline.

ST-25 (Tianshu 天枢)

- Front-Mu point of the Large Intestine.
- On the addomen, 2 cun lateral to the umbilicus.

ST-26 (Wailing 外陵)

- On the lower abdomen, 1 cun below the umbilicus, 2 cun lateral to the anterior midline.

ST-27 (Daju 大巨)

- On the lower abdomen, 2 cun below the umbilicus, 2 cun lateral to the anterior midline.

ST-28 (Shuidao 水道)

- On the lower abdomen, 3 cun below the umbilicus, 2 cun lateral to the anterior midline.

ST-29 (Guilai 归来)

- On the lower abdomen, 4 cun below the umbilicus, 2 cun lateral to the anterior midline.

ST-30 (Qichong 气冲)

- On the lower abdomen, 5 cun below the umbilicus, 2 cun lateral to the anterior midline.

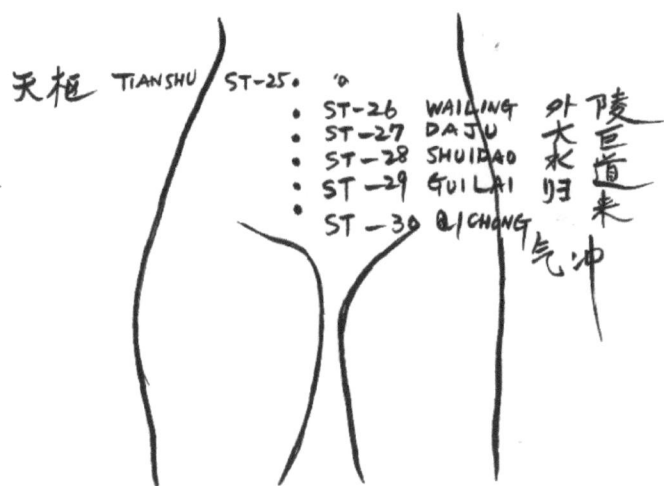

ST-31 (Biguan 髀关)

- On the upper thigh, on the line connecting the anterosuperior iliac spine and the superiolateral border of the patella.

Sitting upright with the knee flexed, two-finger width down directly from the inguinal groove, directing the midline of the patella.

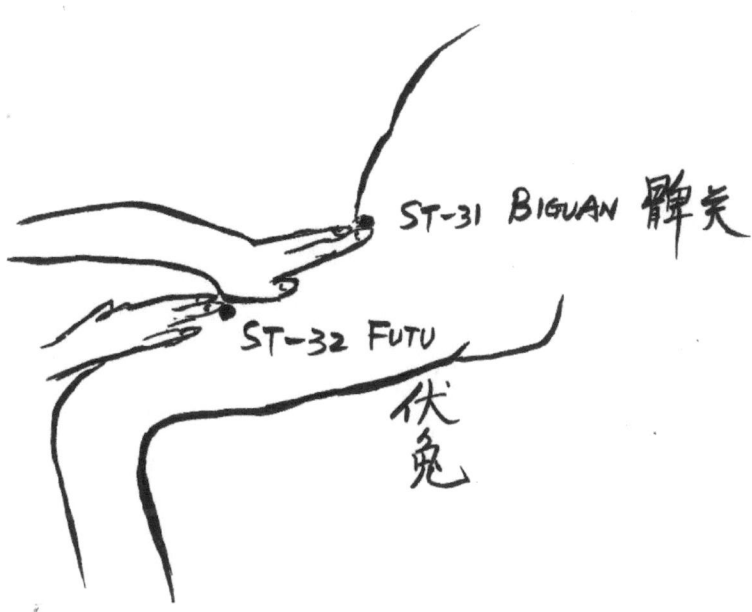

ST-32 (Futu 伏兔)

- On the thigh, on the line connecting anterior superior iliac spine and the lateral border of the patella, 6 cun above the laterosuperior border of the patella.

Sitting upright with the knee flexed, puts the center of the transverse crease of the wrist on the center of the upper border of the patella with closed fingers on the thigh. The point is where the tip of the middle finger.

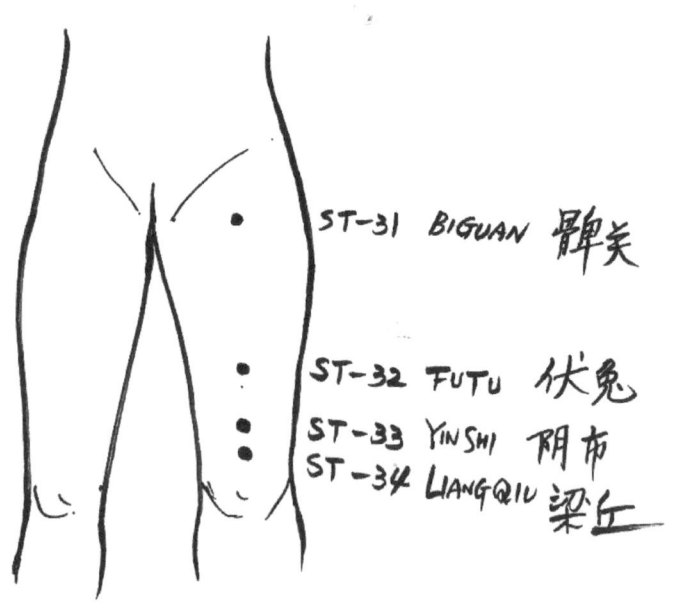

ST-33 (Yinshi 阴市)

- On the thigh, the point is 3 cun above the laterosuperior border of patella. On the line connecting the anterior superior lilac spine and the lateral superior border of the patella.

ST-34 (Liang 梁丘)

- Xi-Cleft point of the Stomach channel.
- On the thigh, 2 cun above the superiolateral border of the patella.

ST-35 (Dubi 犊鼻)

- On the knee, in the depression lateral to the patella and the patellar ligament.

ST-36 (Zusanli 足三里)

- He-Sea point of the Stomach channel.
- 3 cun inferior to ST-35 (Dubi 犊鼻), one finger-breadth (middle finger) lateral to the anterior crest of the tibia.

ST-37 (Shangjuxu 上巨虚)

- Lower He-Sea point of the Large Intestine.
- On the lower leg, 6 cun inferior to ST-35 (Dubi 犊鼻), one finger- breadth (middle finger) lateral to the anterior crest of the tibia.

ST-38 (Tiaokou 条口)

- On the lower leg, 8 cun inferior to ST-35 (Dubi 犊鼻), one finger-breadth (middle finger) lateral to the anterior crest of the tibia.

ST-39 (Xijuxu 下巨虚)

- Lower He-Sea point of the Small Intestine.
- Point of the Sea of Blood.
- On the lower leg, 9 cun inferior to ST-35 (Dubi 犊鼻), one finger- breadth (middle finger) lateral to the anterior crest of the tibia.

ST-40 (Fenglong 丰隆)

- Luo-Connecting point of the Stomach channel.
- On the lower leg, 8 cun superior to the prominence of the lateral malleolus, lateral to ST-38 (Tiaokou 条口), two finger-breadths lateral to the anterior crest of the tibia.

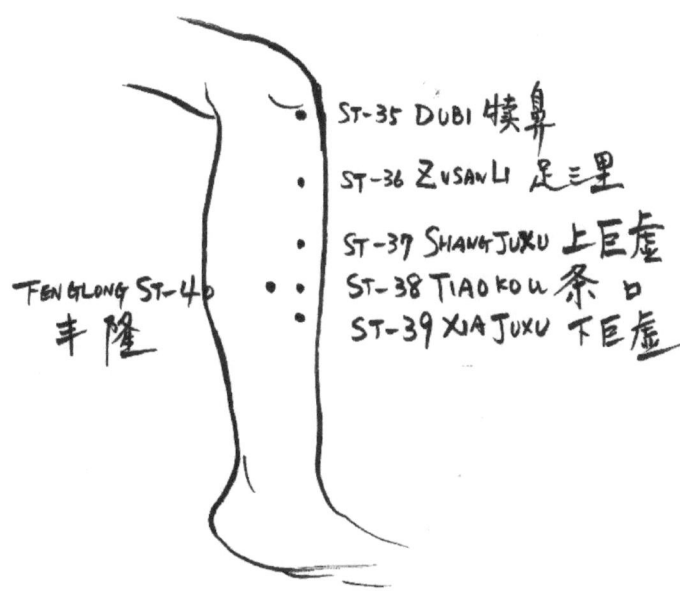

ST-35 DUBI 犊鼻
ST-36 ZUSANLI 足三里
ST-37 SHANGJUXU 上巨虚
ST-38 TIAO KOU 条口
ST-39 XIA JUXU 下巨虚
FENGLONG ST-40 丰隆

ST-41 (Jiexi 解溪)

- Midpoint of the dorsum of the foot at the transverse malleolus, in a depression between the tendons of extensor hallucis longus and extensor digitorum longus.

ST-42 (Chongyang 冲阳)

- Yuan-Source point of the Stomach channel.
- Highest point on the dorsum of the foot, in the depression distal to the junction of the second and third metatarsal bones.

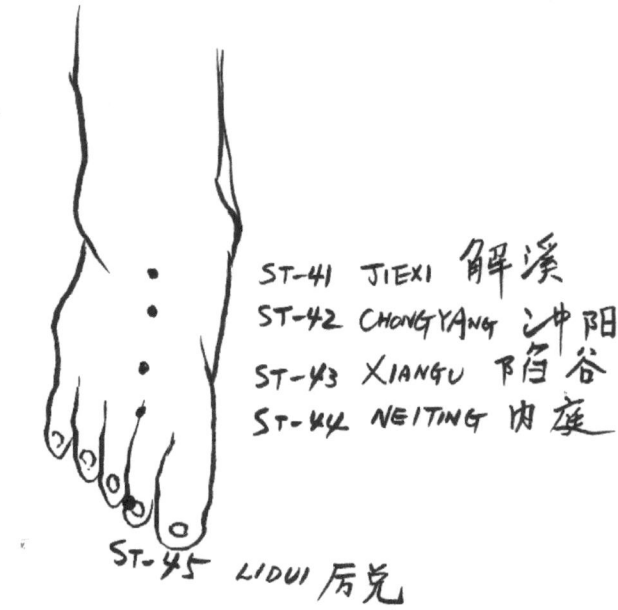

ST-41 JIEXI 解溪
ST-42 CHONGYANG 冲阳
ST-43 XIANGU 陷谷
ST-44 NEITING 内庭
ST-45 LIDUI 厉兑

ST-43 (Xiangu 陷谷)

- On the dorsum of the foot, between the second and third metatarsal bones, 1 cun proximal to ST-44 (Neiting 内庭).

ST-44 (Neiting 内庭)

- On the dorsum of the foot, between the second and third toes, at the end of the vertical skin crease of the web.

ST-45 (Lidui 厉兑)

- On the lateral side of the 2nd toe, 0.1 cun beside the corner of the nail.

V.The Spleen Channel of Foot-Taiyin
足太阴脾经经穴

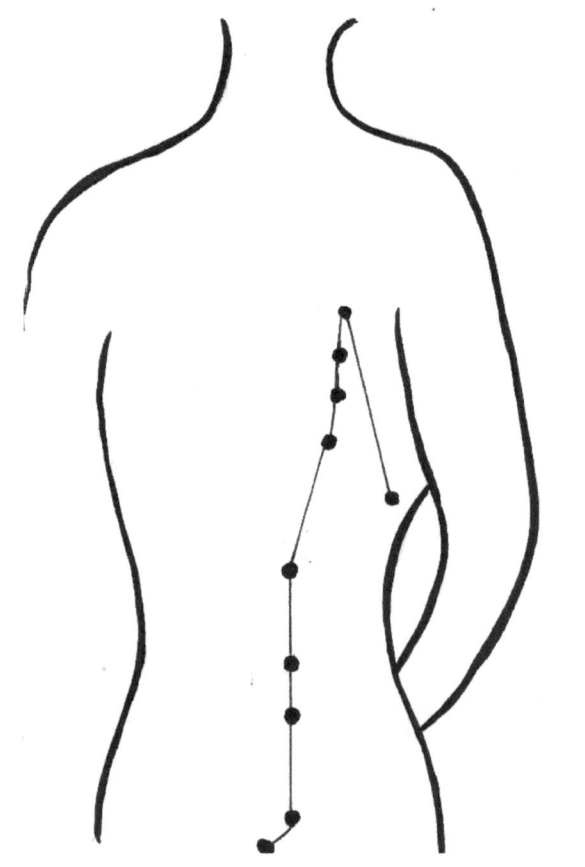

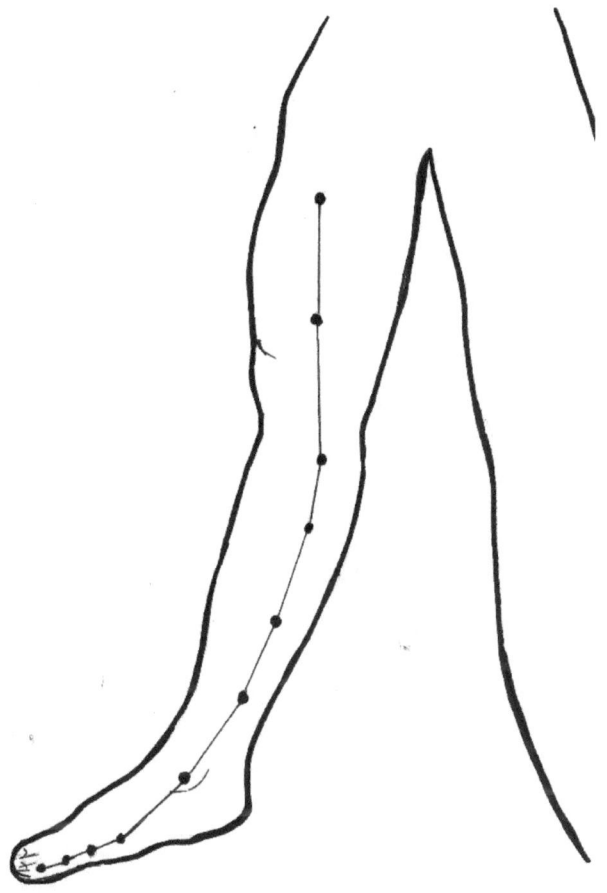

Starts from the tip of the big toe, passing through the anterior medial aspect of the knee and thigh, and enters the abdomen, then up the ribs to a point on the chest below the armpit. It contains 21 different acupoints.

SP-1 (Yinbai 隱白)

- On the medial side of the big toe, 0.1 cun beside the corner of the nail.

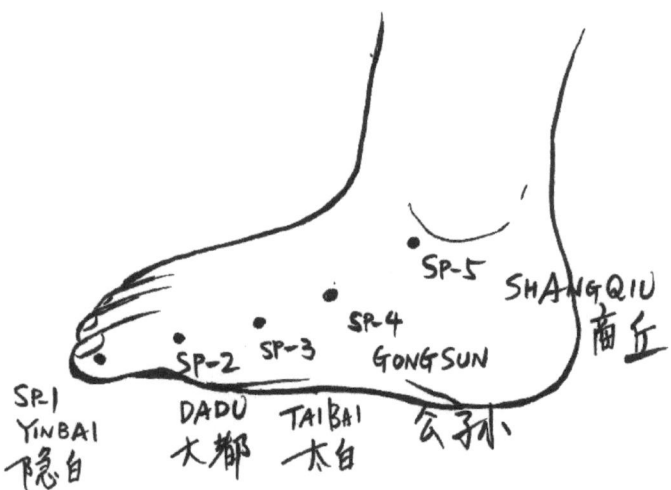

SP-2 (Dadu 大都)

- On the medial side of the big toe, in the depression distal and inferior to the first metatarso-phalangeal joint.

SP-3 (Taibai 太白)

- Yuan -Source point of the Spleen channel.

- On the medial side of the foot, in the depression proximal and inferior to the first metatarso-phalangeal joint.

SP-4 (Gongsun 公孙)

- Luo-Connecting point of the Spleen channel.
- On the medial side of the foot, in the depression distal and inferior to the base of the first metatarsal bone.

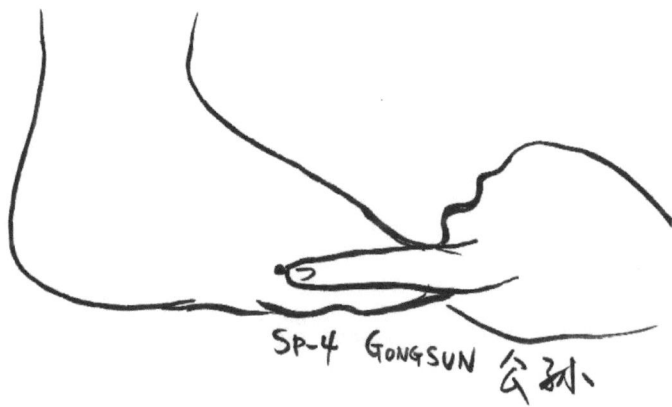

SP-4 GONGSUN 公孙

SP-5 (Shangqiu 商丘)

- On the medial side of the foot, in the depression distal and inferior to the medial malleolus, the midpoint.

SP-6 (Sanyinjiao 三阴交)

- 3 cun directly above the tip of medial malleolus, in the depression near the posterior border of the tibia.

SP-7 (Lougu 漏谷)

- 6 cun above the tip of the medial malleolus, og 3 cun superior to SP-6 (Sanyinjiao 三阴交), in a depression posterior to to the medial crest of the tibia.

SP-8 (Diji 地机)

- Xi-Cleft point of the Spleen channel.
- 3 cun below SP-9 (Yinlingquan 阴陵泉), on the line connecting the tip of the medial malleolus.

SP-9 (Yinlingquan 阴陵泉)

- He-Sea point of the Spleen channel.
- On the medial side of the lower leg, in a depression posterior and inferior to the medial condyle to the tibia.

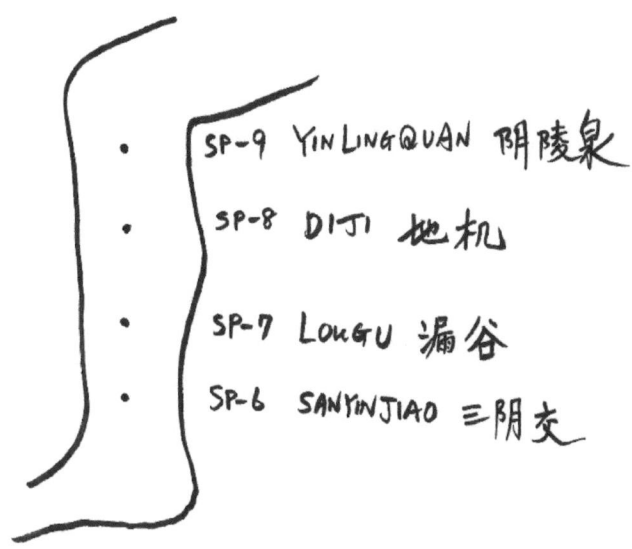

SP-10 (Xuehai 血海)

- Sea of Blood.
- When the knee is flexed, 2 cun above medial border of the patella, directly above SP-9 (Yinlingquan 阴陵泉).

When the knee is flexed, put the palm on the upper border of the patella with four fingers directed upward, and the thumb forming an angle of 45 degrees with the index finger. The point is where the tip of the thumb.

SP-11 (Jimen 箕门)

- On the medial side of the thigh, 6 cun above SP-10 (Xuehai 血海).

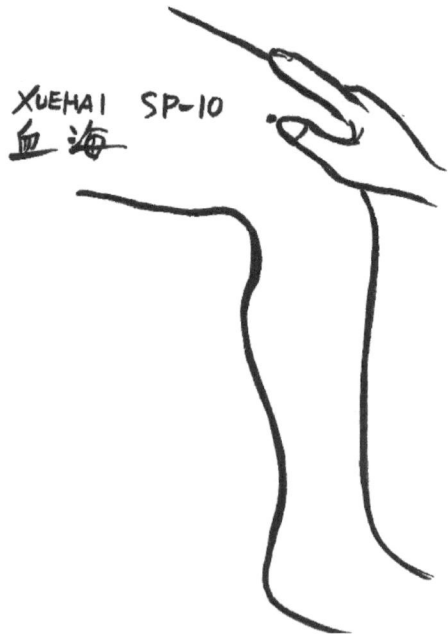

SP-12 (Chongmen 冲门)

- 6 cun above SP-10 (Xuehai 血海), 3.5 cun lateral to the midpoint of the upper border of the symphysis pubis.

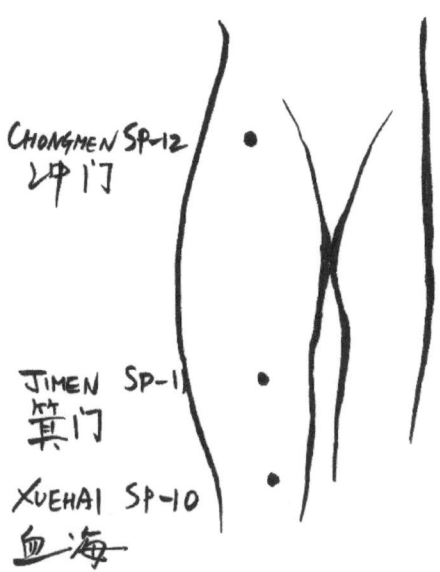

CHONGMEN SP-12
冲门

JIMEN SP-11
箕门

XUEHAI SP-10
血海

SP-13 (Fushe 府舍)

- On the lower abdomen, 0.7 cun superior to SP-12 (Chongmen 冲门), 4 cun lateral to the midline.

SP-14 (Fujie 腹結)

- On the lower abdomen, 3 cun above SP-13 (Fushe 府舍).

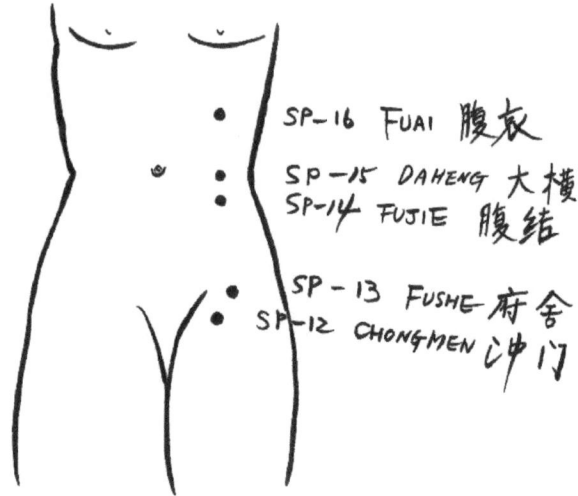

SP-16 FUAI 腹哀
SP-15 DAHENG 大横
SP-14 FUJIE 腹结
SP-13 FUSHE 府舍
SP-12 CHONGMEN 冲门

SP-15 (Daheng 大横)

- On the abdomen, 4 cun lateral to the center of the umbilicus.

SP-16 (Fuai 腹哀)

- On the abdomen, 3 cun above the umbilicus, 4 cun lateral to the anterior midline.

SP-17 (Shidou 食窦)

- On the lateral side of the chest, in the fifth intercostal space, 6 cun lateral to the anterior midline.

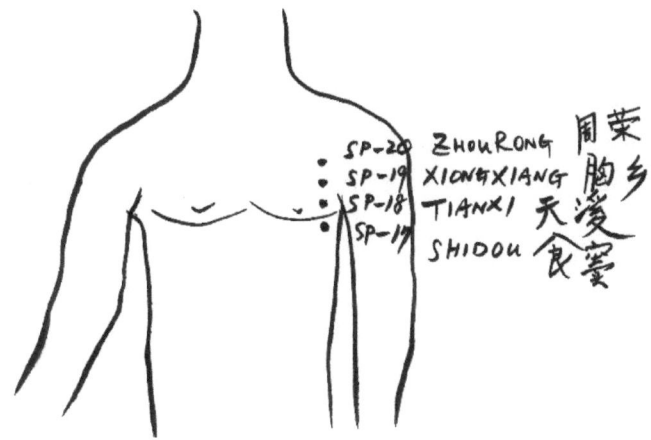

SP-18 (Tianxi 天溪)

- On the lateral side of the chest, in the fourth intercostal space, 6 cun lateral to the anterior midline.

SP-19 (Xiongxiang 胸乡)

- On the lateral side of the chest, in the third intercostal space, 6 cun lateral to the anterior midline.

SP-20 (Zourong 周荣)

- On the lateral side of the chest, in the second intercostal space, 6 cun lateral to the midline.

SP-21 (Dabao 大包)

- Great Luo-Connecting point of the Spleen.
- On the lateral side of the chest, in the middle axillary line, in the sixth intercostal space.

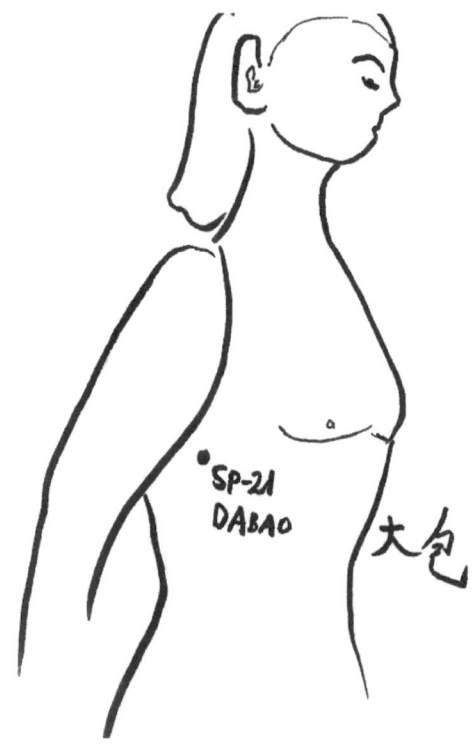

V. The Heart Channel of Hand-Taiyang
手阴心经经穴

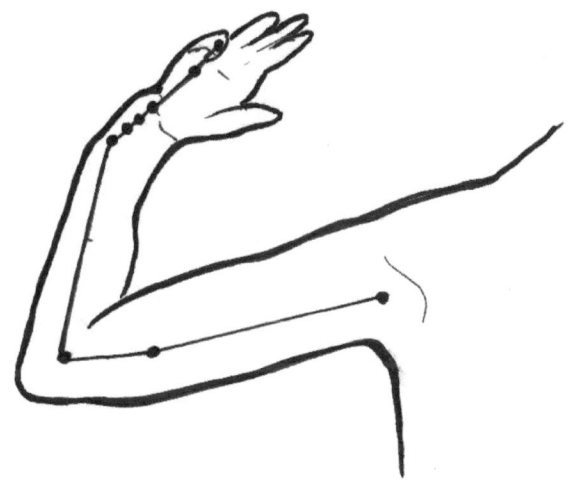

Starts in the armpit, passing through the forearm to the pisiform region proximal to the palm, then follows to the tip of the little finger. It contains 9 different acupoints.

HT-1 (Jiquan 极泉)

- When raise the arm, the point in the depression at the centre of the axilla.

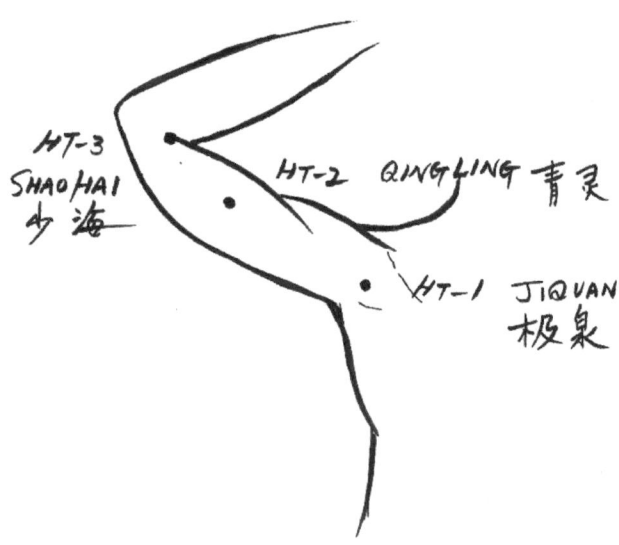

HT-2 (Qingling 青灵)

- 3 cun above the medial end of the transverse cubital crease, on the line connecting HT-1 (Jiquan 极泉) and HT-3 (Shaohai 少海).

HT-3 (Shaohai 少海)

- He-Sea point of the Heart channel.
- When the elbow is flexed, at the midpoint of the line jointing the medial end of the transverse cubital crease.

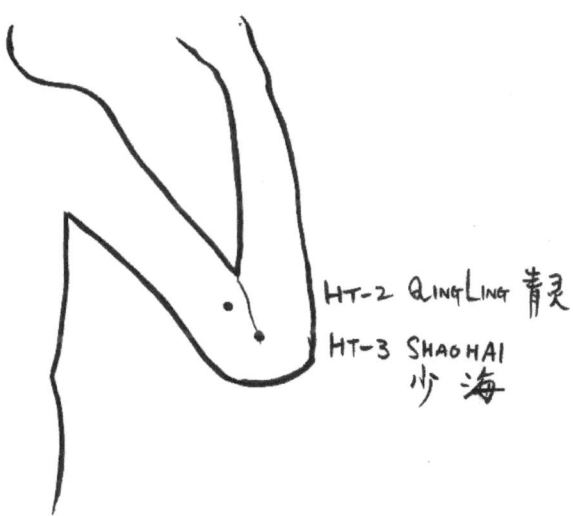

HT-2 QingLing 青灵
HT-3 Shaohai 少海

HT-4 (Lingdao 灵道)

- On the palm side of the forearm, 1.5 cun above the transverse crease of the wrist.

HT-5 (Tongli 通里)

- Luo-Connecting point of the Heart channel.
- On the palm side of the forearm, 1 cun above the transverse crease of the wrist.

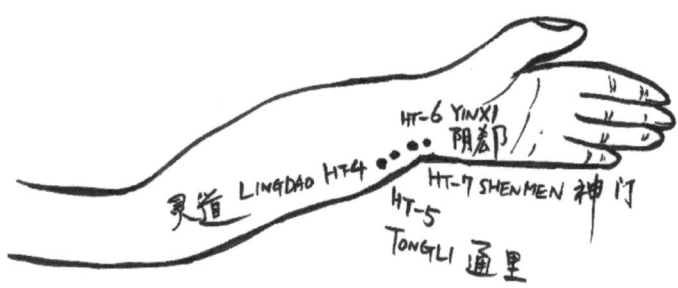

HT-6 (Yinxi 阴郄)

- Xi-Cleft point of the Heart channel.
- On the palmer side of the forearm, 0.5 cun above the transverse crease of the wrist.

HT-7 (Shenmen 神门)

- Yuan-Source of the Heart channel.
- At the ulnar end of the transverse crease of the wrist, on the radial side of flexor carpi ulnaris, in the depression at the proximal border of the pisform bone.

HT-8 (Shaofu 少府)

- On the palm, in the depression between the fourth and fifth metacarpal bones. When a fist is made, the point is on where the tip of the little finger rests.

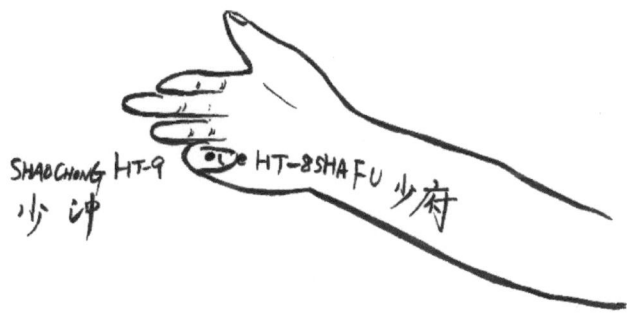

HT-9 (Shaochong 少冲)

- On the radial side of the little finger, 0.1 cun beside the corner of the nail.

VI. The Small Intestine Channel of Hand-Taiyang 手太阳小肠经经穴

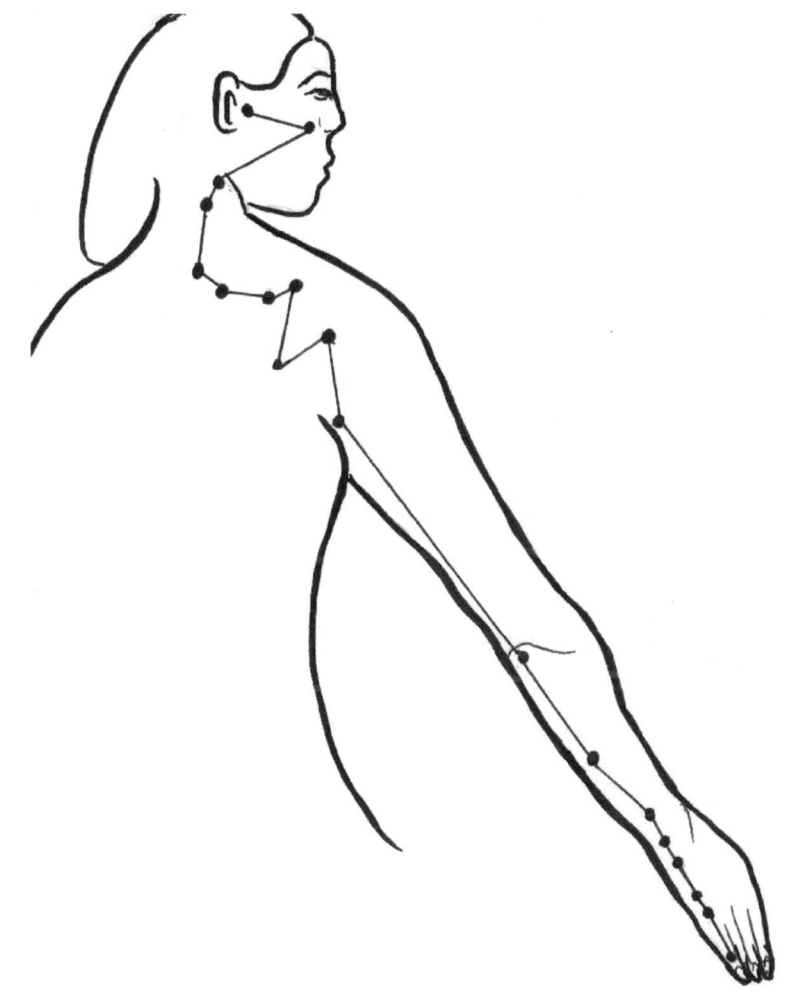

Starts from the ulnar side of the tip of the little finger and follows the ulnar side of the dorsum of the hand to the wrist, passing through the arm to the shoulder blade to the neck, then up to the eye and across to the ear. It contains 19 different acupoints.

SI-1 (Shaoze 少泽)

- On the ulnar side of the little finger, 0.1 cun from the corner of the nail.

SI-2 (Qiangu 前谷)

- When a loose fist is made, the point on the ulnar end of the crease, side of the 5th metacarpophalangeal joint.

SI-3 (Houxi 后溪)

- When a loose fist is made, the point on the ulnar side of the hand, at the end of the transverse crease proximal to the fifth metacarpophalangeal joint.

SI-4 (Wangu 腕骨)

- Yuan-Source point of the Small Intestine Channel.

- On the ulnar side of the hand, in the depression between the base of the fifth metacarpal bone and the triquetral bone.

SI-5 (Yanggu 阳谷)

- At the ulnar side of the wrist, in the depression between styloid process of the ulna and the triquetral bone.

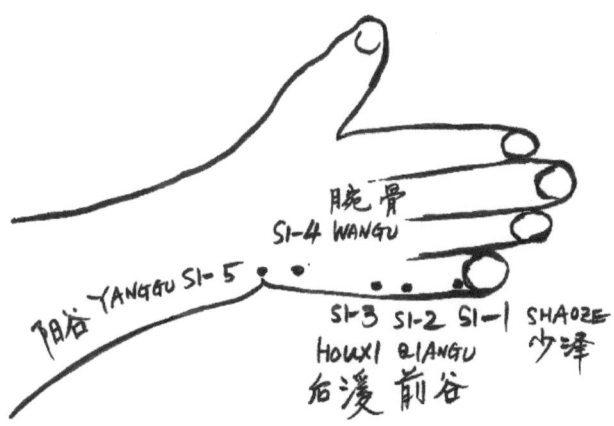

SI-6 (Yanglao 养老)

- Xi-Cleft point of the Small Intestine channel.
- With the palm facing downward, put a fingertip on the highest spot of the head of ulna, in a depression under the finger, on the radial side of the styloid process of the ulna.

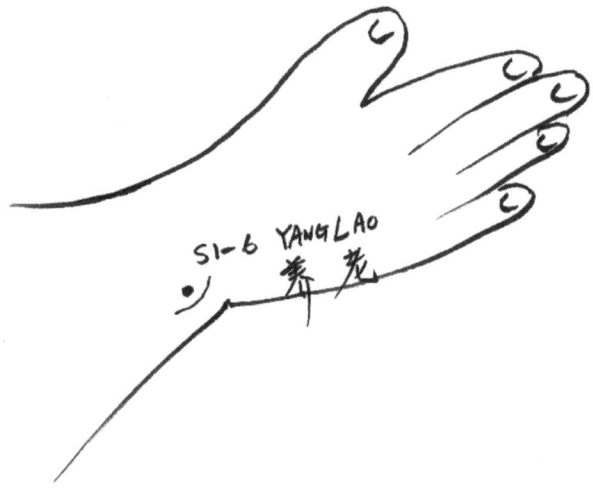

SI-7 (Zhizheng 支正)

- Luo-connecting point of the Small Intestine channel.

- On the line connecting SI-6 (Yanglao 养老) and SI-8(Xiaohai 小海), 5 cun proximal to the dorsal crease of the wrist.

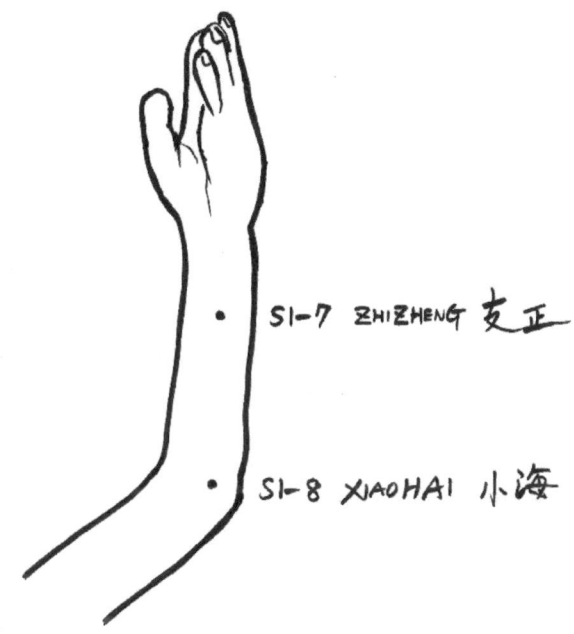

SI-8(Xiaohai 小海)

- He-Sea point of the Small Intestine channel.
- When the elbow is flexed, in the depression between the olecranon of the ulna and the tip of the medial epicondyle of the humerus.

SI-9 (Jianzhen 肩贞)

- On the shoulder, posterior and inferior to the shoulder joint. 1 cun above the posterior end of the axillary fold.

SI-10 (Naoshu 臑俞)

- On the shoulder, above the posterior end of the axillary fold, in the depression below the lower border of the scapular spine.

SI-11 (Tianzong 天宗)

- On the scapula, in the depression of the center of the subscapular fossa, at the same level of the fourth thoracic vertebra.

SI-12 (Bingfeng 秉风)

- On the scapra, in the centre of the suprascapular fossa, directly above SI-11 (Tianzong 天宗), in a dipression found when the arm is lifted,

SI-13 (Quyuan 曲垣)

- On the chest, in the fourth intercostal space, at the corner of the nipple, 4 cun lateral to the anterior midline.

.SI-14 (Jianwaishu 肩外俞)

- 3 cun lateral to the lower border of the spinous process of the 1st thoracic vertebra.

SI-15 (Jianzhongshu 肩中俞)

- 2 cun lateral to DU-14 (Dazhui 大椎).

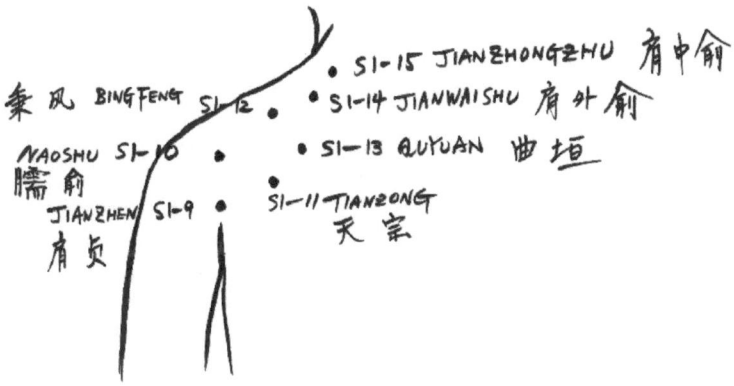

SI-16 (Tianchuang 天窗)

- Posterior border of the sternocleido-mastoid muscle level with the laryngeal prominence.

SI-17 (Tianrong 天容)

- Posterior to the angle of the mandible, in the depression on the anterior border of the sternocleidomastoid muscle.

SI-18 (Quanliao 顴髎)

- Directly below the outer canthus, in the depression of the lower border of the zygomatic bone.

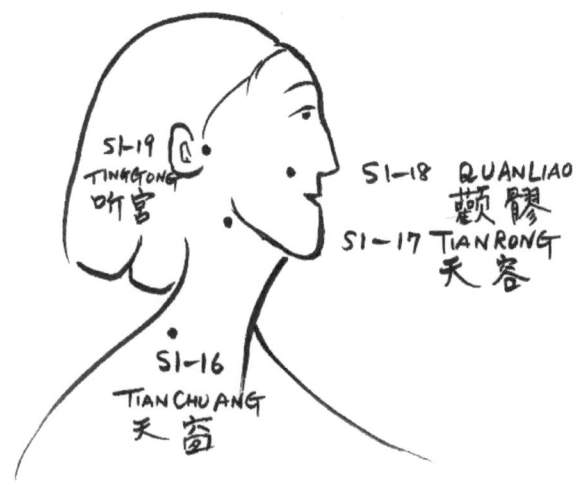

SI-19 (Tinggong 听宫)

- In the depression formed when the mouth is open. Anterior to the tragus and posterior to the condyloid process of the mandible.

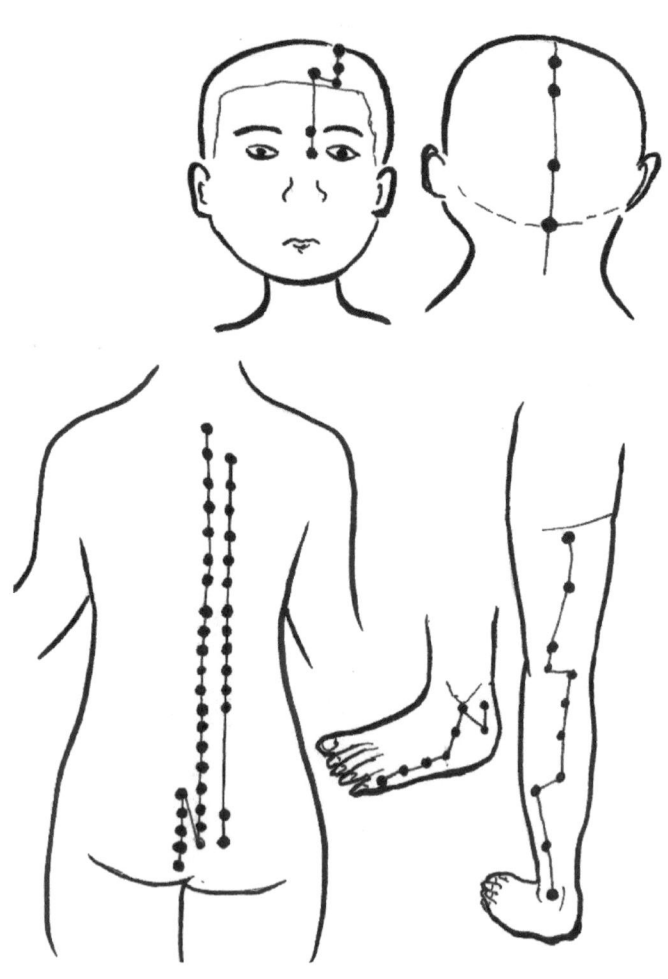

VII. The Bladder channel of Foot-Taiyang
足太阳膀胱经经穴

Starts in the eye and ascending to the forehead and over the top of the skull. It splits below the hairline in back. One branch passes through down the shoulder blade and down to the middle of the low back. The other one passes downward to the outside of the spine through down the back of the leg to the heel. It contains 67 different acupuncture points.

BL-1 (Jingming 睛明)

- On the closed eye, in the depression slightly above, 0.1 cun lateral and superior to the inner canthus.

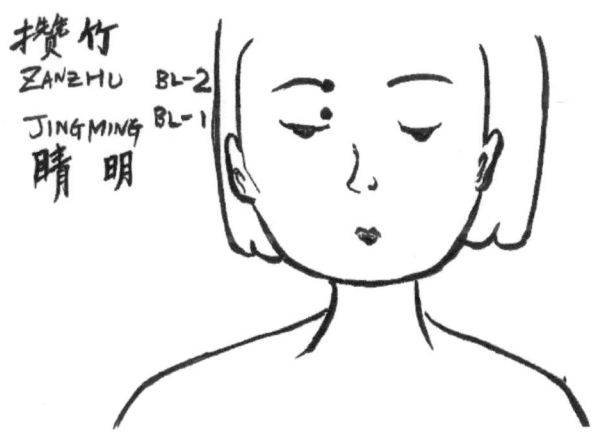

BL-2 (Cuanzhu 攒竹)

- On the face, directly above BL-1 (Jingming 睛明), in the depression on the medial end of the eyebrow.

BL-3 (Meichong 眉冲)

- On the head, directly above BL-2 (Zanzhu 攒竹), 0.5 cun above the anterior hairline.

BL-4 (Qucha 曲差)

- On the head, 0.5 cun above the anterior hairline, 1.5 cun lateral to the midline.

BL-5 (Wuchu 五处)

- On the head, 1 cun directly above the midway of the anterior hairline, 1.5 cun lateral to the anterior midline.

BL-6 (Chengguang 承光)

- On the head, 2.5 cun directly above the midway of the anterior hairline, 1.5 cun lateral to the anterior midline.

BL-7 (Tongtian 通天)

- On the head, 4 cun directly above the midway of the anterior hairline, 1.5 cun lateral to the anterior midline.

BL-8 (Louque 络却)

- On the head, 5.5 cun directly above the midway of the anterior hairline, 1.5 cun lateral to the anterior midline.

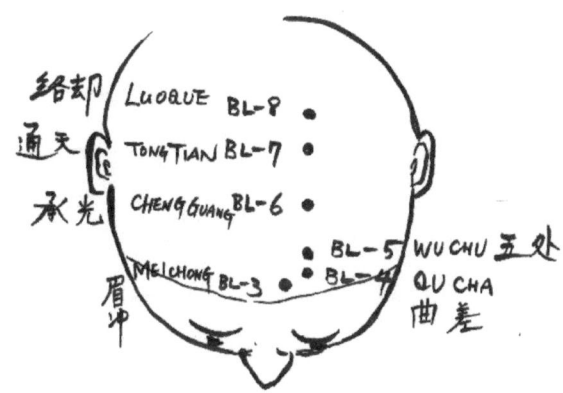

BL-9 (Yuzhen 玉枕)

- On the occiput, 2.5 cun directly above the midpoint of the posterior hairline and 1.3 cun lateral to the midline, in the depression on the level of the upper border of the external occipital protuberance.

BL-10 (Tianzhu 天杼)

- 1.3 cun lateral to the midpoint of the posterior hairline, in the depression on the lateral border of the trapezius muscle.

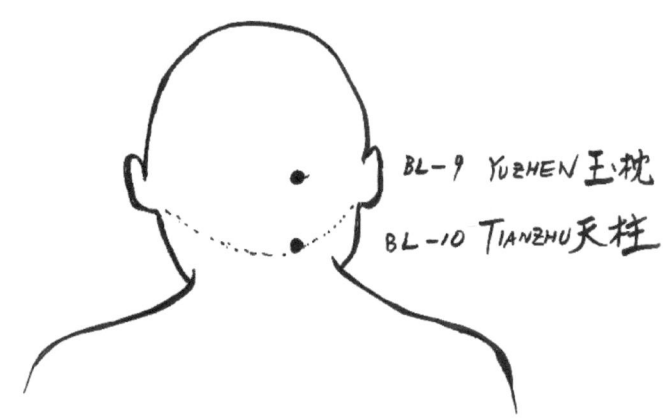

BL-9 YUZHEN 玉枕

BL-10 TIANZHU 天柱

BL-11 (Dazhu 大杼)

- Point of the Sea of Blood.
- On the back, below the spinous process of the first thoracic vertebra (T1), 1.5 cun lateral to the posterior midline.

BL-12 (Fengmen 风门)

- On the back, below the spinous process of the second thoracic vertebra (T2), 1.5 cun lateral to the posterior midline.

BL-13 (Feishu 肺俞)

- Back-Shu point of the Lung.
- On the back, below the spinous process of the third thoracic vertebra (T3), 1.5 cun lateral to the posterior midline.

BL-14 (Jueyinshu 厥阴俞)

- Back-Shu point of the Pericardium.
- On the back, below the spinous process of the fourth thoracic vertebra (T4), 1.5 cun lateral to the posterior midline.

BL-15 (Xinshu 心俞)

- Back-Shu point of the Heart.
- On the back, below the spinous process of the fifth thoracic vertebra (T5), 1.5 cun lateral to the posterior midline.

BL-16 (Dushu 督俞)

- On the back, below the spinous process of the sixth thoracic vertebra (T6), 1.5 cun lateral to the posterior midline.

BL-17 (Geshu 膈俞)

- On the back, below the spinous process of the seventh thoracic vertebra (T7), 1.5 cun lateral to the posterior midline.

BL-18 (Ganshu 肝俞)

- Back-Shu point of the Liver.
- On the back, below the spinous process of the ninth thoracic vertebra (T9), 1.5 cun lateral to the posterior midline.

BL-19 (Danshu 胆俞)

- Back-Shu point of the Gall Bladder.
- On the back, below the spinous process of the tenth thoracic vertebra (T10), 1.5 cun lateral to the posterior midline.

BL-20 (Pishu 脾俞)

- Back-Shu point of the Spleen.
- On the back, below the spinous process of the eleventh thoracic vertebra (T11), 1.5 cun lateral to the posterior midline.

BL-21 (Weishu 胃俞)

- Back-Shu point of the Stomach.
- On the back, below the spinous process of the twelfth thoracic vertebra (T12), 1.5 cun lateral to the posterior midline.

BL-22 (Sanjiaoshu 三焦俞)

- Back-Shu point of the Sanjiao.
- On the lower back, below the spinous process of the first lumbar vertebra (L1), 1.5 cun lateral to the posterior midline.

BL-23 (Shenshu 肾俞)

- Back-Shu point of the Kidneys.
- On the lower back, below the spinous process of the second lumbar vertebra (L2), 1.5 cun lateral to the posterior midline.

BL-24 (Qihaishu 气海俞)

- Sea of Qi Shu.
- On the lower back, below the spinous process of the third lumbar vertebra (L3), 1.5 cun lateral to the posterior midline.

BL-25 (Dachangshu 大肠俞)

- Large Intestine Shu
- On the lower back, below the spinous process of the fouth lumbar vertebra (L4), 1.5 cun lateral to the posterior midline.

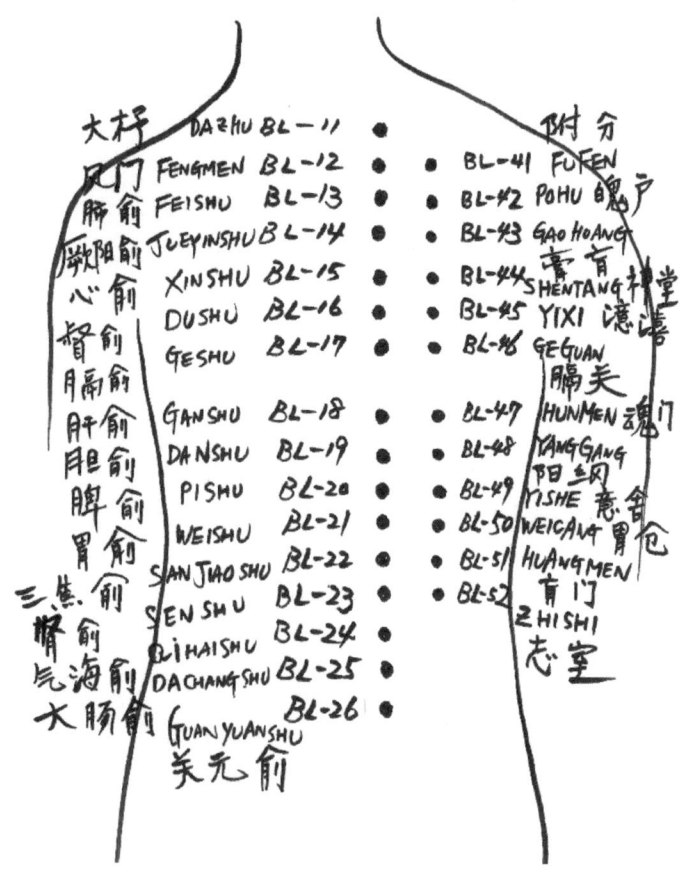

BL-26 (Guanyuanshu 关元俞)

- Gate of the Origin Shu.
- On the lower back, below the spinous process of the fifth lumbar vertebra (L5), 1.5 cun lateral to the posterior midline.

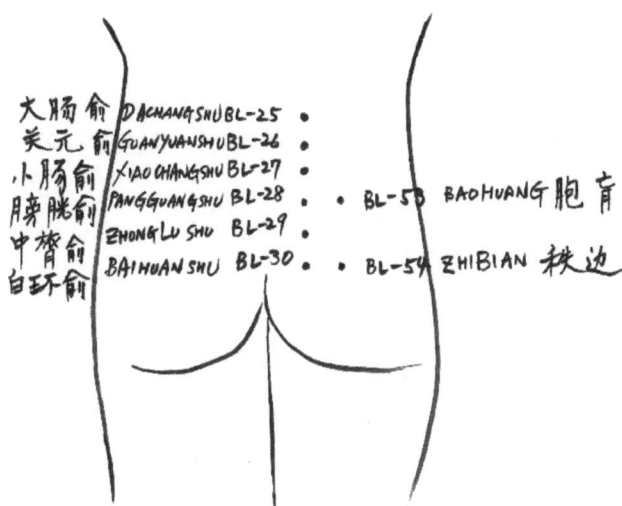

BL-27 (Xiaochangshu 小肠俞)

- Back-Shu point of the Small Intestine.
- On the sacrum, 1.5 cun lateral to the midline, at the level of the first posterior sacral foramen.

BL-28 (Pangguangshu 膀胱俞)

- Back-Shu point of the Bladder.
- On the sacrum, 1.5 cun lateral to the midline, at the level of the second posterior sacral foramen.

BL-29 (Zhonglushu 中膂)

- Mid-Spine Shu.
- On the sacrum, 1.5 cun lateral to the midline, at the level of the third posterior sacral foramen.

BL-30 (Baihuanshu 白环俞)

- White Ring Shu.
- On the sacrum, 1.5 cun lateral to the midline, at the level of the fourth posterior sacral foramen.

BL-31 (Shangliao 上髎)

- On the sacrum, first posterior sacral foramen.

BL-32 (Ciliao 次髎)

- On the sacrum, second posterior sacral foramen.

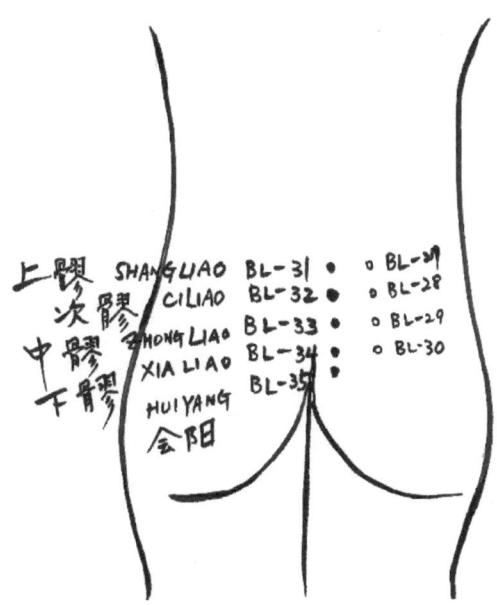

BL-33 (Zhongliao 中髎)

- On the sacrum, third posterior sacral foramen.

BL-34 (Xialiao 下髎)

- On the sacrum, fourth posterior sacral foramen.

BL-35 (Huiyang 会阳)

- 0.5 cun lateral to the tip of the coccyx.

BL-36 (Chengfu 承扶)

- On the midpoint of the transverse gluteal fold, the point in the middle of the back of the thigh.

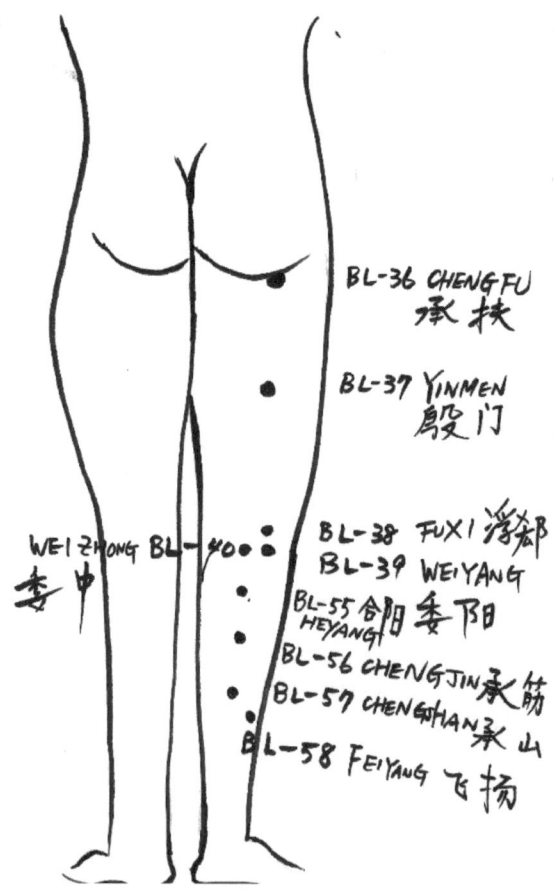

BL-37 (Yinmen 殷门)

- On the back of the thigh, 6 cun directly below BL-36 (Chengfu 承扶).

BL-38 (Fuxi 浮郄)

- On the back of the knee, 1 cun above BL-39 (Weiyang 委阳), on the medial side of the tendon of biceps femoris on the lateral side of the popliteal fossa.

BL-39 (Weiyang 委阳)

- Lower He-Sea point of the Sanjiao.
- On the back of the knee, at the lateral end of the popliteal crease, on the medial border of the tendon of biceps femoris.

BL-40 (Weizhong 委中)

- He-Sea point of the Bladder channel.
- On the back of the knee, on the midpoint of the transverse crease of the popliteal fossa.

BL-41 (Fufen 附分)

- On the back, below the spinous process of the second thoracic vertebra (T2), 3 cun lateral to the midline and level with BL-12 (Fengmen 风门).

BL-42 (Pohu 魄户)

- On the back, below the spinous process of the third thoracic vertebra (T3), 3 cun lateral to the midline and level with BL-13 (Feishu 肺俞).

BL-43 (Gaohuangshu 膏肓俞)

- On the back, below the spinous process of the fourth thoracic vertebra (T4), 3 cun lateral to the midline and level with BL-14 (Jueyinshu 厥阴俞).

BL-44 (Shentang 神堂)

- On the back, below the spinous process of the fifth thoracic vertebra (T5), 3 cun lateral to the midline and level with BL-15 (Xinshu 心俞).

BL-45 (Yixi 噫嘻)

- On the back, below the spinous process of the sixth thoracic vertebra (T6), 3 cun lateral to the midline and level with BL-16 (Dushu 督俞).

BL-46 (Geguan 膈关)

- On the back, below the spinous process of the seventh thoracic vertebra (T7), 3 cun lateral to the midline and level with BL-17 (Geshu 膈俞).

BL-47 (Hunmen 魂门)

- On the back, below the spinous process of the ninth thoracic vertebra (T9), 3 cun lateral to the midline and level with BL-18 (Ganshu 肝俞).

BL-48 (Yanggang 阳刚)

- On the back, below the spinous process of the tenth thoracic vertebra (T10), 3 cun lateral to the midline and level with BL-19 (Danshu 胆俞).

BL-49 (Yishe 意舍)

- On the back, below the spinous process of the eleventh thoracic vertebra (T11), 3 cun lateral to the midline and level with BL-20 (Pishu 脾俞).

BL-50 (Weicang 胃仓)

- On the back, below the spinous process of the twelfth thoracic vertebra (T12), 3 cun lateral to the midline and level with BL-21 (Weishu 胃俞).

BL-51 (Huangmen 肓门)

- On the lower back, below the spinous process of the first lumber vertebra (L1), 3 cun lateral to the midline and level with BL-22 (Sanjiaoshu 三焦俞).

BL-52 (Zhishi 志室)

- On the lower back, below the spinous process of the second lumber vertebra (L2), 3 cun lateral to the midline and level with BL-23 (Shenshu 肾俞).

BL-53 (Baohuang 包肓)

- On the buttock, 3 cun lateral to the midline, level with the second posterior sacral foramen.

BL-54 (Zhibian 秩边)

- On the buttock, 3 cun lateral to the midline, level with the fourth posterior sacral foramen.

BL-55 (Heyang 合阳)

- On the posterior side of the leg, 2 cun directly below to BL-40 (Weizhong 委中).

BL-56 (Chengjin 承筋)

- On the lower leg, 5 cun below BL-40 (Weizhong 委中), in the centre of the belly of gastrocnemius muscle.

BL-57 (Chengshan 承山)

- On the lower leg, 8 cun below BL-40 (Weizhong 委中), midway between BL-40 (Weizhong 委中) and BL-60 (Kunlun 昆仑).

BL-58 (Feiyang 飞扬)

- Luo-connecting point of the Bladder channel.
- On the lower leg, 7 cun directly above BL-60 (Kunlun 昆仑).

BL-59 (Fuyang 跗阳)

- On the lower leg, 3 cun directly above BL-60 (Kunlun 昆仑).

BL-60 (Kunlun 昆仑)

- Behind the ankle joint, in the depression between the prominence of the lateral malleolus.

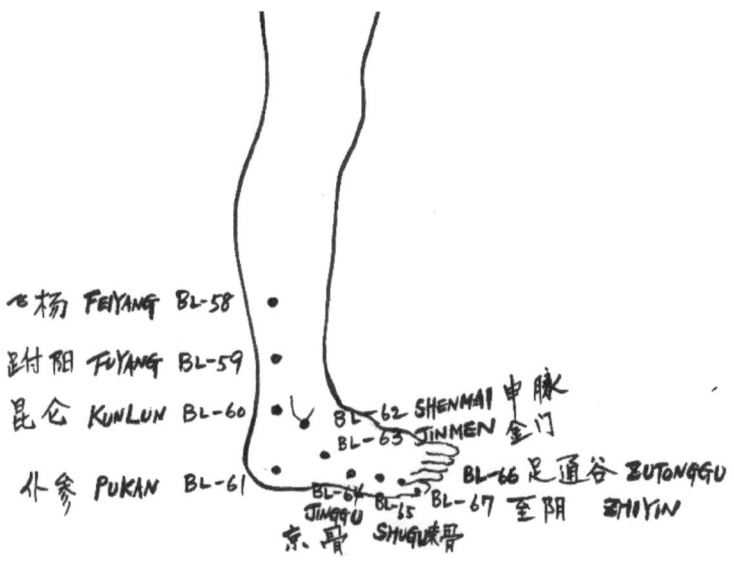

BL-61 (Pucan 仆参)

- On the lateral side of the foot, directly below BL-60 (Kunlun 昆仑).

BL-62 (Shenmai 申脉)

- On the lateral side of the foot, directly below the lateral malleolus.

BL-63 (Jinmen 金门)

- Xi-Cleft point of the Bladder channel.
- On the lateral side of the foot, in the depression below the cuboid bone which lies between the heel bone and the tuberosity of the 5th metatarsal bone.

BL-64 (Jinggu 京骨)

- Yuan-Source point of the Bladder channel.
- On the lateral side of the foot, in the depression below the tuberosity of the 5th metatarsal bone.

BL-65 (Shugu 束骨)

- On the lateral side of the foot, posterior to the fifth metatarsal bone.

BL-66 (Zutonggu 足通谷)

- On the lateral side of the foot, anterior to the fifth metatarso-phalangeal bone.

BL-67 (Zhiyin 至阴)

- On the lateral side of the small toe, about 0.1 cun from the corner of the nail.

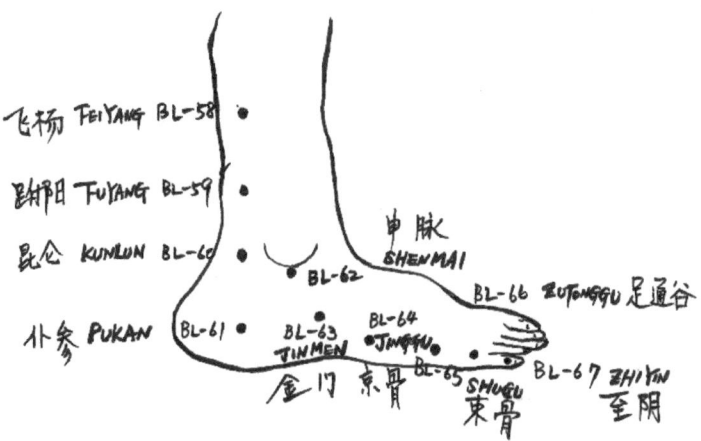

VIII. The Kidney Channel of Foot-Shaoyin 足少阴肾经经穴

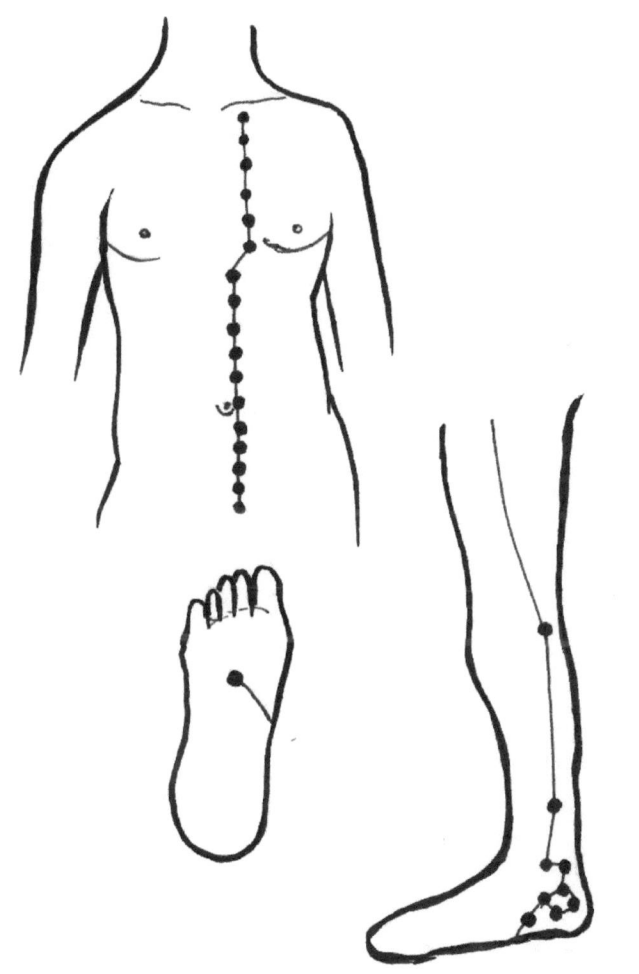

Starts in the arch of the foot and, ascends along the medial side of the leg and to the side of the midline of the abdomen and chest. It contains 27 different acupupoints.

KI-1 (Yongquan 涌泉)

- On the sole, at the junction of the anterior one-third and posterior two thirds of the sole, between the second and third metatarsal bones.

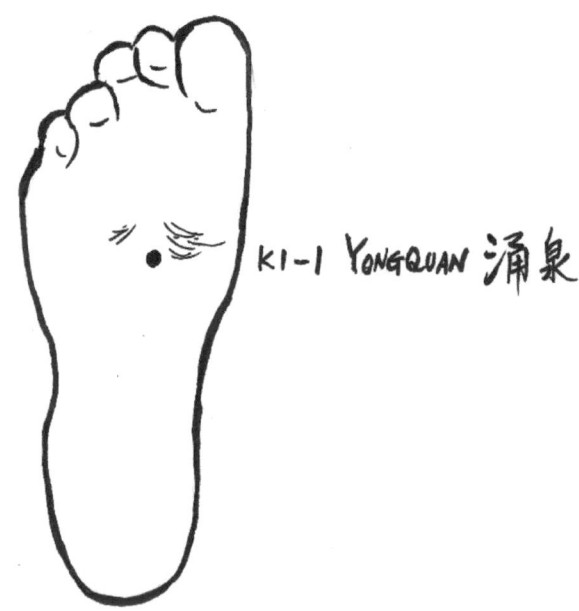

KI-2 (Rangu 然谷)

- Anterior and inferior to the medial malleolus, in the depression on the lower border of the tuberosity of the navicular bone.

KI-3 (Taixi 太溪)

- Yuan-Source of the Kidney channel.
- On the medial malleolus, in the depression between the prominence of the medial malleolus and the Achilles tendon.

KI-4 (Dazhong 大钟)

- Luo-Connecting point of the Kidney channel.
- 0.5 cun below posterior to KI-3 (Taixi 太溪), on the anterior border of the medial side of the tendon calcaneus.

KI-5 (Shuiquan 水泉)

- Xi-Cleft point of the Kidney channel.
- 1 cun directly below KI-3 (Taixi 太溪), in the depression of the medial side of the tuberosity of the calcaneum.

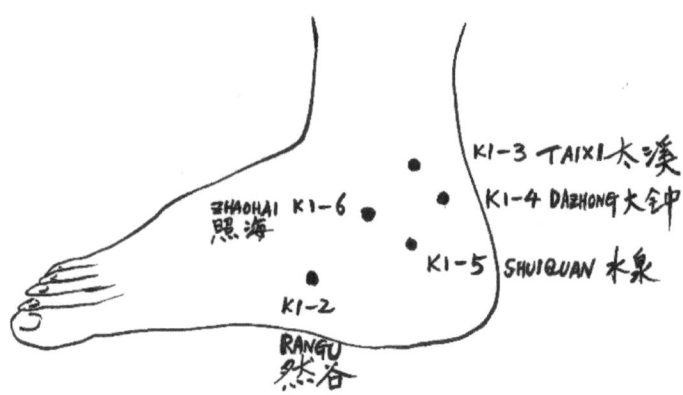

KI-6 (Zhaohai 照海)

- 1 cun below the prominence of the medial malleolus.

KI-7 (Fuliu 复瘤)

- On the medial side of the foot, 2 cun superior to KI-3 (Taixi 太溪) anterior to the Achilles tendon.

KI-8 (Jiaoxin 交信)

- On the medial side of the lower leg, 2 cun above KI-3 (Taixi 太溪), 0.5 cun anterior to KI-7 (Fuliu 复瘤).

KI-9 (Zhubin 筑宾)

- On the medial border of the lower leg, 5 cun superior to KI-3 (Taixi 太溪), on the line connecting KI-3 (Taixi 太溪) and KI-10 (Yingu 阴谷).

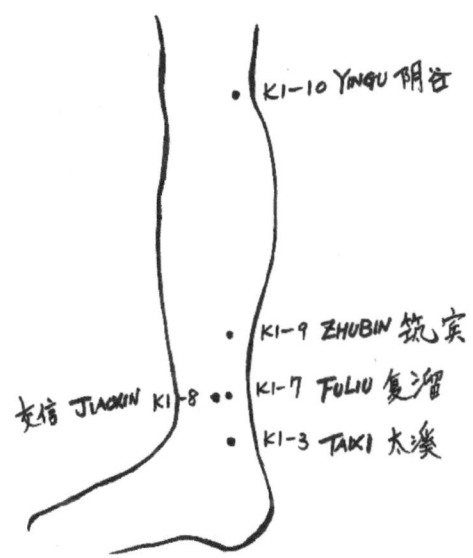

KI-10 (Yingu 阴谷)

- He-Sea point of the Kidney channel.
- On the medial end of the popliteal crease, when the knee is flexed, the point is at the medial side of the transverse popliteal fossa.

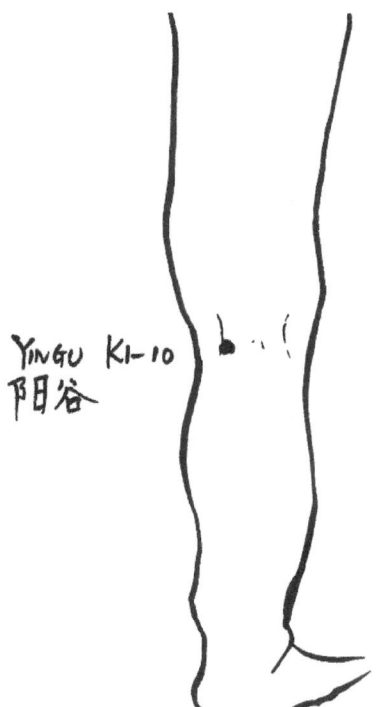

YINGU KI-10
阴谷

KI-11 (Henggu 横骨)

- On the lower abdomen, 5 cun below the umbilicus, 0.5 cun lateral to the anterior midline.

KI-12 (Dahe 大赫)

- On the lower abdomen, 4 cun below the umbilicus, 0.5 cun lateral to the anterior midline.

KI-13 (Qixue 气穴)

- On the lower abdomen, 3 cun below the umbilicus, 0.5 cun lateral to the anterior midline.

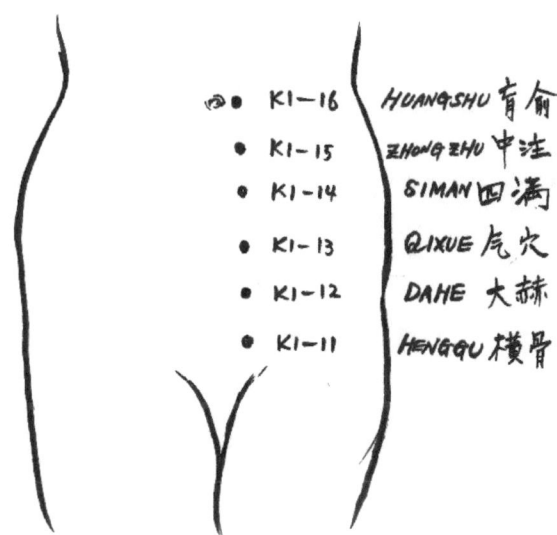

KI-14 (Siman 四满)

- On the lower abdomen, 2 cun below the umbilicus, 0.5 cun lateral to the anterior midline.

KI-15 (Zhongzhu 中注)

- On the lower abdomen, 1 cun below th umbilicus, 0.5 cun lateral to the anterior midline.

KI-16 (Huangshu 肓俞)

- On the middle abdomen, 0.5 cun lateral to the center of the umbilicus.

KI-17 (Shangqu 商曲)

- On the upper abdomen, 2 cun above the umbilicus, 0.5 cun lateral to the anterior midline.

KI-18 (Shiguan 石关)

- On the upper abdomen, 3 cun above the umbilicus, 0.5 cun lateral to the anterior midline.

KI-19 (Yindu 阴都)

- On the upper abdomen, 4 cun above the umbilicus, 0.5 cun lateral to the anterior midline.

KI-20 (Futonggu 腹通谷)

- On the upper abdomen, 5 cun above the umbilicus, 0.5 cun lateral to the anterior midline.

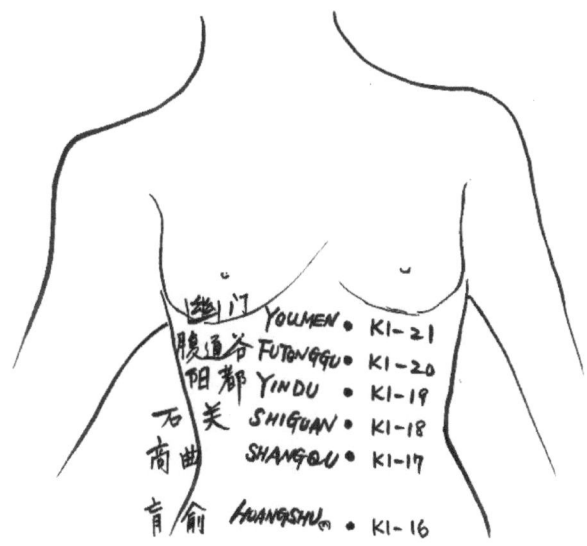

KI-21 (Youmen 幽门)

- On the upper abdomen, 6 cun above the umbilicus, 0.5 cun lateral to the midline.

KI-22 (Bulang 步廊)

- On the chest, in the fifth intercostal space, 2 cun lateral to the midline.

KI-23 (Shenfeng 神封)

- On the chest, in the fourth intercostal space, and 2 cun lateral to the anterior midline.

KI-24 (Lingxu 灵墟)

- On the chest, in the third intercostal space, and 2 cun lateral to the anterior midline.

KI-25 (Shencang 神藏)

- On the chest, in the second intercostal space, and 2 cun lateral to the anterior midline.

KI-26 (Yuzhong 彧中)

- On the chest, in the first intercostal space, and 2 cun lateral to the anterior midline.

KI-27 (Shufu 俞府)

- On the chest, below the lower border of the clavicle, 2 cun lateral to the midline.

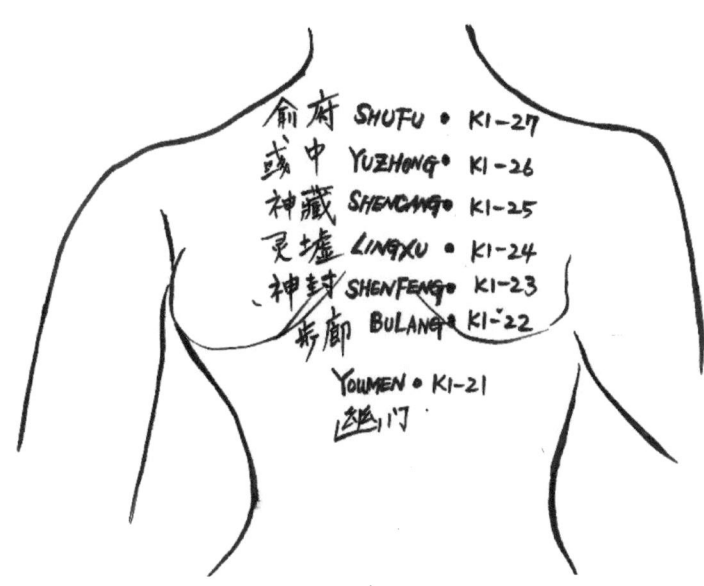

俞府 SHUFU • KI-27
彧中 YUZHONG • KI-26
神藏 SHENCANG • KI-25
灵墟 LINGXU • KI-24
神封 SHENFENG • KI-23
步廊 BULANG • KI-22

YOUMEN • KI-21
幽门

IX. The Pericardium Channel of Hand-Yueyin 手蕨阴心包经经穴

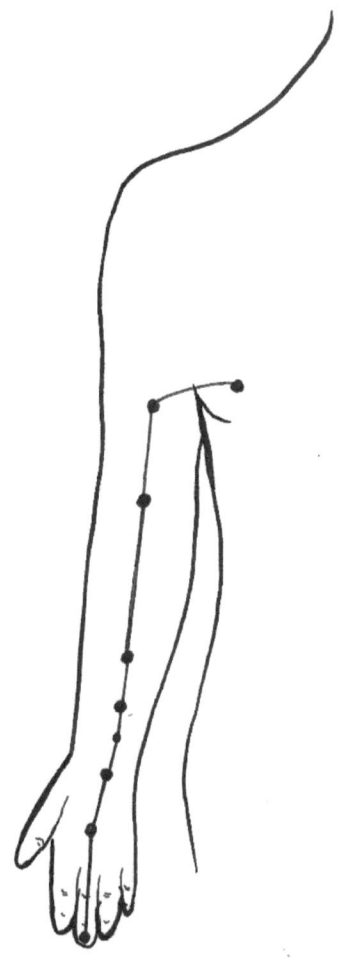

Originates from the chest, the side of the nipple through the armpit and down the arm to the tip of the middle finger. It contains 9 different acupoints.

P-1 (Tianchi 天池)

- On the chest, in the fourth intercostal space, 1 cun lateral to the nippe, and 5 cun lateral to the anterior midline.

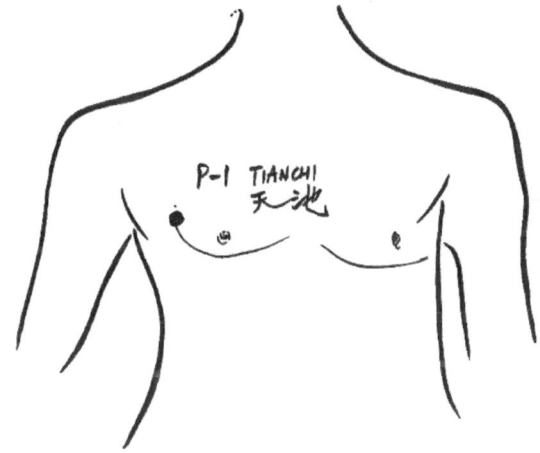

P-2 (Tianquan 天泉)

- On the medial side of the arm, 2 cun below the axillary fold, between the two heads of biceps brachii.

P-3 (Quze 曲泽)

- He-Sea point of the Pericardium channel.
- At the midpoint of the transverse cubital crease, at the ulnar side of the tendon of biceps brachii.

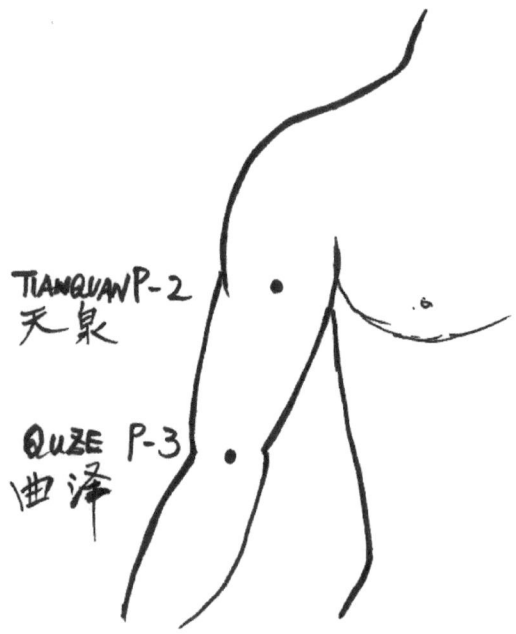

P-4 (Ximen 郄门)

- On the palmar side of the forearm, 5 cun above the transverse crease of the wrist, on the line connecting P-3 (Quze 曲泽) and P-7 (Daling 大陵), between the tendons of palmaris longus and flexor carpi radialis.

P-5 (Jianshi 间使)

- On the palmar side of the forearm, 3 cun above the transverse crease of the wrist, on the line connecting P-3 (Quze 曲泽) and P-7 (Daling 大陵), between the tendons of palmaris longus and flexor carpi radialis.

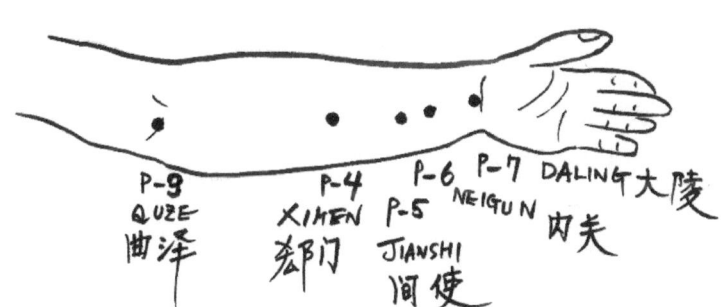

P-6 (Neiguan 内关)

- Luo-Connecting point of the Pericardium channel.
- On the palmar side of the forearm, 2 cun above the transverse crease of the wrist, on the line connecting P-3 (Quze 曲泽) and P-7 (Daling 大陵), between the tendons of palmaris longus and flexor carpi radialis.

P-7 (Daling 大陵)

- Yuan-Source of the Pericardium channel.
- On the palmar side of the forearm, at the midpoint of the transverse crease of the wrist, between the tendons of palmaris longus and flexor carpi radialis.

P-8 (Laogong 劳宫)

- On the palm, between the second and third metacarpal bones. When the fist is made, the point is below the tip of the middle finger.

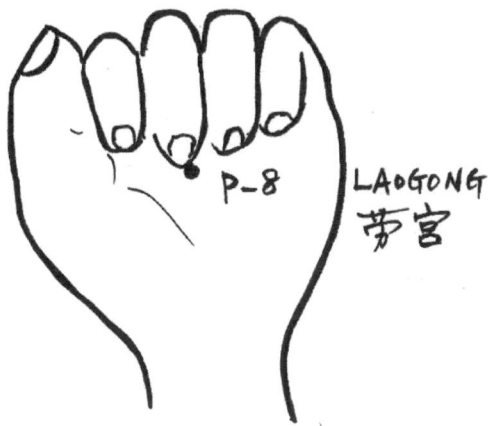

P-9 (Zhongchong 中冲)

- At the center of the tip of the middle finger.

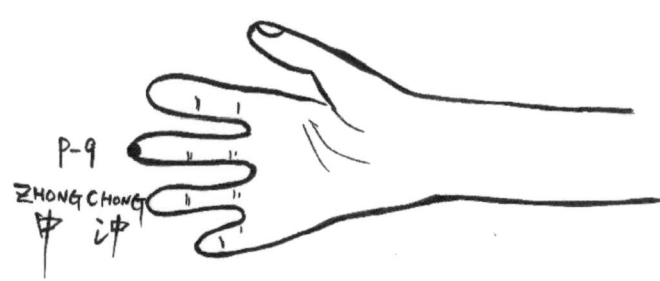

X. The Sanjiao Channel of Hand-Shaoyang 手少阳三焦经经穴

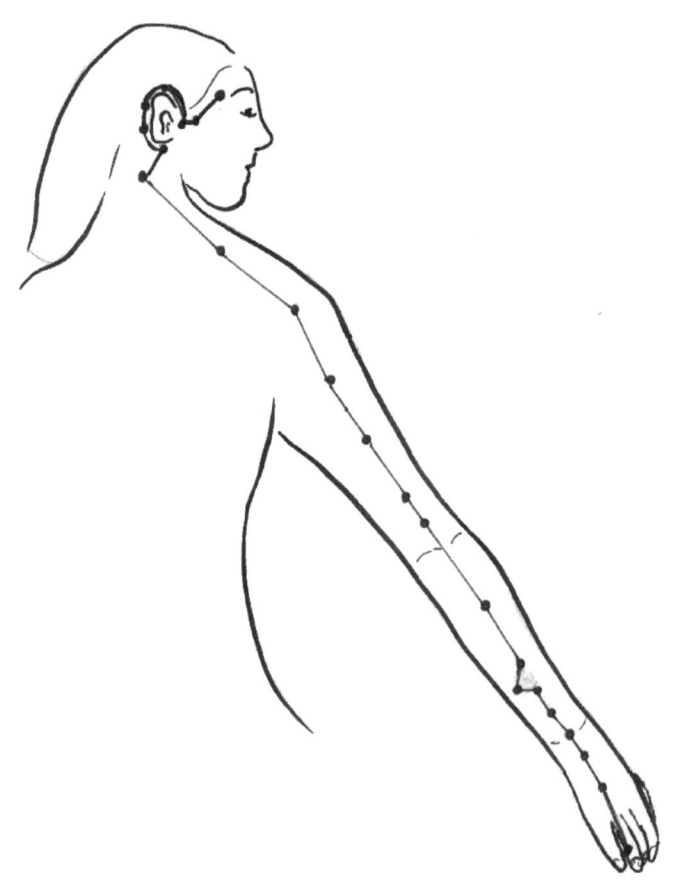

Originates from the tip of the ring finger, runs upward the dorsal aspect of the forearm to the shoulder region and ascends to the neck to the ear, then across the forehead, downward to the cheek to the end of the eyebrow. It contains 23 different acupoints.

SJ-1 (Guanchong 关冲)

- On the ulnar side of the ring finger, 0.1 cun beside the corner of the nail.

SJ-2 (Yemen 液门)

- When the fist is clenched, between the ring and little fingers, proximal to the margin of the web.

SJ-3 (Zhongzhu 中诸)

- On the dorsum of the hand between the fourth and fifth the metacarpal bones, in the depression proximal to the metacarpophalangeal joint, 1 cun posterior to SJ-2 (Yemen 液门).

SJ-4 (Yangchi 阳池)

- Yuan-Source point of the Sanjiao channel.

- On the dorsum of the wrist, in the depression between the tendons of extensor digitorum communis and extensor digiti minimi.

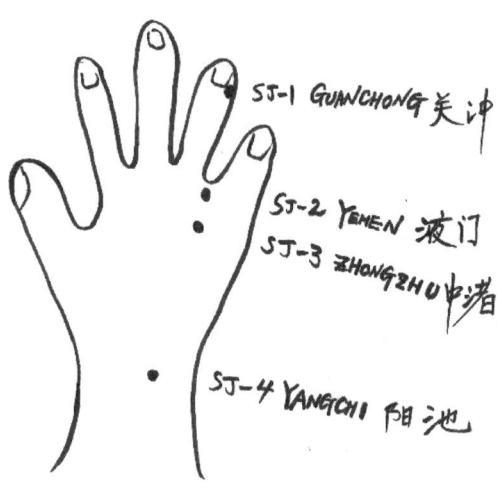

SJ-5 (Waiguan 外关)

- Luo-Connecting point of the Sanjiao channel.
- On the dorsum of the forearm, on the line connecting SJ-4 (Yangchi 阳池) and olecranon, 2 cun proximal to the dorsal crease of the wrist, between the radius and the ulna.

SJ-6 (Zhigou 支沟)

- On the dorsum of the forearm, on the line connecting SJ-4 (Yangchi 阳池) and olecranon, 3 cun proximal to the dorsal crease of the wrist, between the radius and the ulna.

SJ-7 (Huizong 会宗)

- Xi-Cleft point of the Sanjiao channel.
- On the dorsum of the forearm, at the same level with SJ-6 (Zhigou 支沟), on the radial border of the ulna.

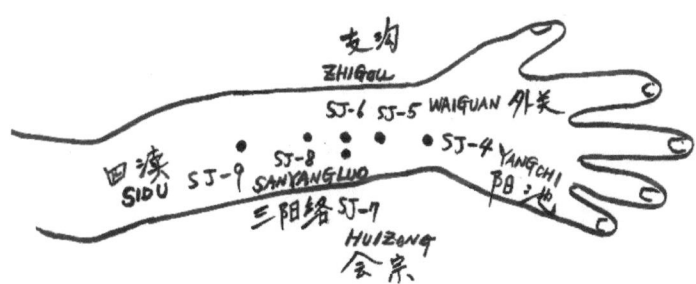

SJ-8 (Sanyangluo 三阳络)

- On the dorsum of the forearm, 4 cun above the transverse crease, between the ulna and the radius.

SJ-9 (Sidu 四读)

- On the dorsum of the forearm, 7 cun proximal to SJ-4 (Yangchi 阳池), in the depression between the radius and the ulna.

SJ-10 (Tianjing 天井)

- He-Sea point of the sanjiao channel.
- With the elbow flexed, in the depression 1 cun proximal to the tip of the olecranon.

SJ-11 (Qinglengyuan 请冷渊)

- With the elbow flexed, 1 cun proximal to SJ-10 (Tianjing 天井).

SJ-12 (Xiaoluo 消泺)

- On the upper arm, on the line connecting SJ-10 (Tianjing 天井) and SJ-14 (Jianliao 肩髎), 4 cun proximal to SJ-10 (Tianjing 天井).

SJ-13 (Naohui 臑会)

- On the lateral side of the upper arm, on the line connecting the tip of the olecranon and SJ-14 (Jianliao 肩髎), 3 cun below SJ-14 (Jianliao 肩髎).

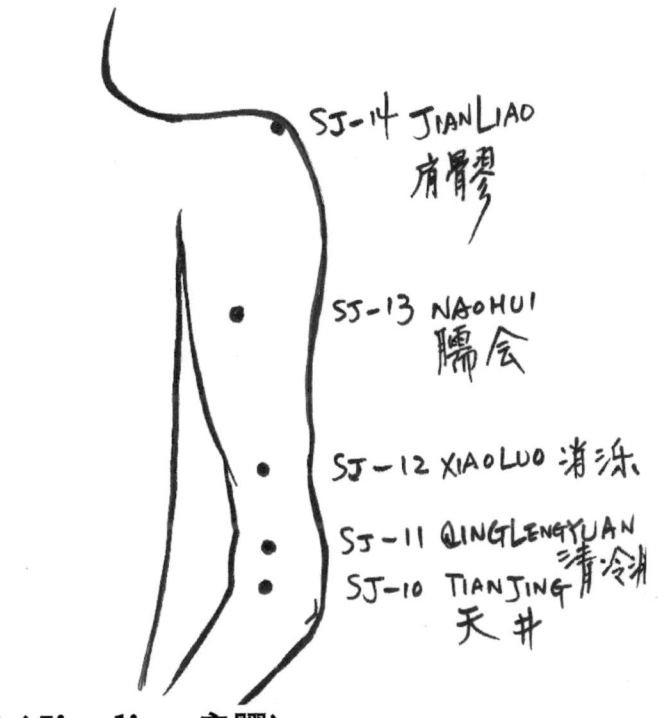

SJ-14 (Jianliao 肩髎)

- On the posterior side of the shoulder, posterior to SJ-14 (Jianliao 肩髎), the point is in the depression inferior and posterior to the acromion when the arm is abducted.

SJ-15 (Tianliao 天髎)

- On the spapula, midway between GB-21 (Jianjing 肩井) and SI-13 (Quyuan 曲垣), 1 cun below GB-21 (Jianjing 肩井).

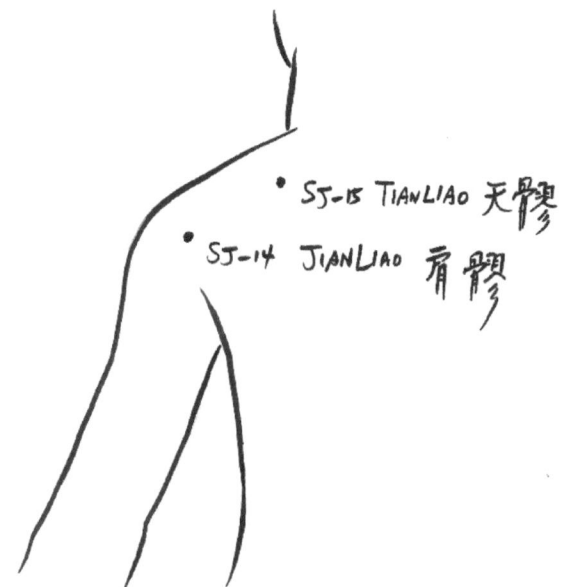

SJ-16 (Tianyou 天牖)

- On the lateral side of the neck, directly below the posterior border of the mastoid process.

On the level of the mandibular angle, on the posterior border of the sternocleidomastoid muscle, 1 cun inferior to GB-12 (Wangu 完骨).

SJ-17 (Yifeng 翳风)

- Behind the earlobe, in the depression between the mandible and mastoid process.

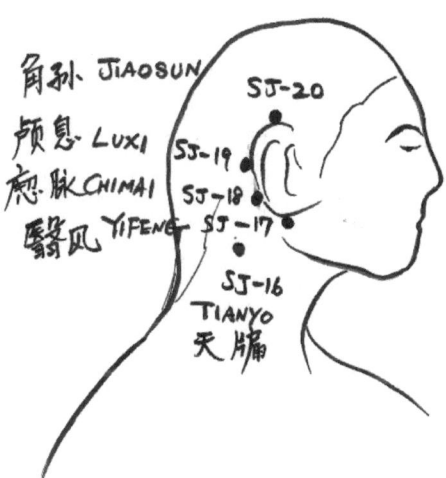

SJ-18 (Chimai 瘈脉)

- On the head, in the depression on the mastoid bone, at the junction of the middle third and lower third of the distance, along the curve of the ear helix from SJ-17 (Yifeng 翳风) to SJ-20 (Jiaosun 角孙), and divide this curved line into three equal parts, and form four points.

SJ-19 (Luxi 颅息)

- On the head, at the junction of the upper and middle third of the curv formed by SJ-17 (Yifeng 翳风) and SJ-20 (Jiaosun 角孙) behind the felix.

SJ-20 (Jiaosun 角孙)

- Directly above the ear apex, within the hair line.

SJ-21 (Ermen 耳门)

- On the face, anterior to the supratragic notch, with the mouth open, the point is in the depression superior to the condyloid process of the mandible.

SJ-22 (Erheliao 耳和髎)

- On the lateral side of the head, the point is the intersection of the level line from the upper border of the root of ear forward and the posterior border of the hairline of the temple.

SJ-23 (Sizhukong 丝竹空)

- In the depression at the lateral end of the eyebrow.

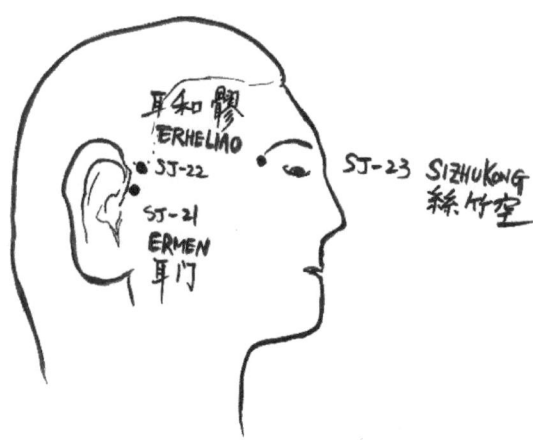

XI. The Gallbladder Channel of Foot-Shaoyang 足少阳胆经经穴

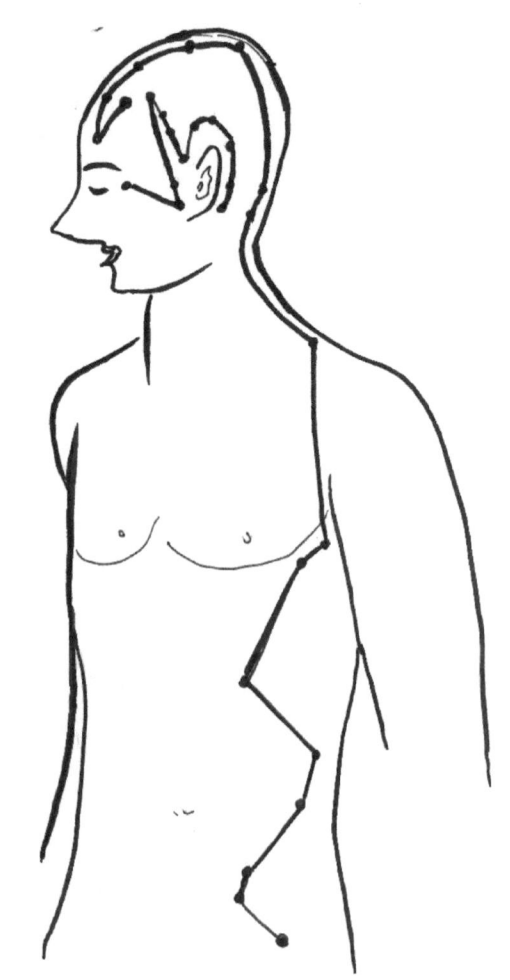

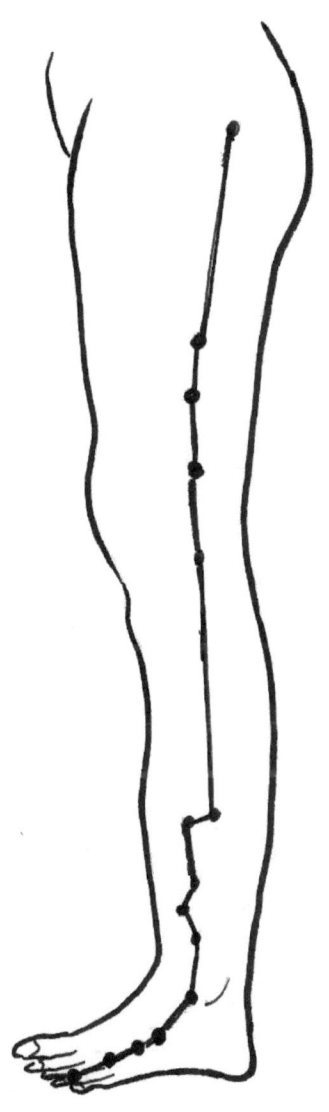

Originates from outer canthus, ascends to the corner of the forehead, back and forth across the skull and then runs down the neck across the shoulder and zigzags back and forth across the chest and abdomen. From there it descends along the lateral aspect of the thigh to the knee, and reaches the anterior aspect of the externa malleolus, and then follow to the tip of the fourth toe. It contains 44 different acupoints.

GB-1 (Tongziliao 瞳子髎)

- 0.5 cun lateral to the outer canthus, in the depression lateral to the orbit.

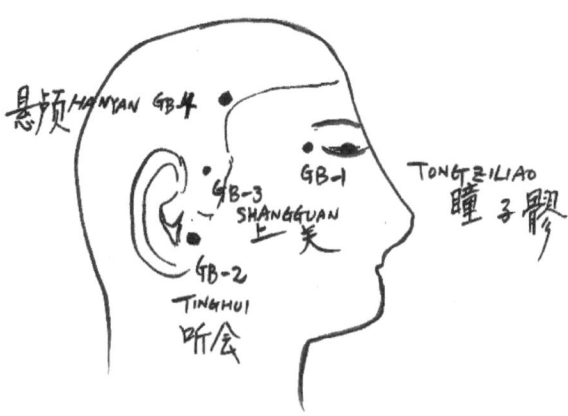

GB-2 (Tinghui 听会)

- On the face, anterior to the intertragic notch. When the mouth is opened, the point is located in a depression appeared.

GB-3 (Shangguan 上关)

- Anterior to the ear, in a depression above the upper border of the zygomatic arch.

GB-4 (Hanyan 頷厌)

- In the temporal region, within the hairline, at the junction of the upper ¼ and lower ¾ of the curved line linking ST-8 (Touwei 头维) and GB-7 (Qubin 曲鬓).

GB-5 (Xuanlu 悬颅)

- In the temporal region, within the hairline, at the midpoint of the curved line connecting ST-8 (Touwei 头维) and GB-7 (Qubin 曲鬓).

GB-6 (Xuanli 悬厘)

- In the temporal region, within the hairline, at the junction of the upper ¾ and lower ¼ of the curved line connecting ST-8 (Touwei 头维) and GB-7 (Qubin 曲鬓).

GB-7 (Qubin 曲鬓)

- In the temporal region, within the hairline, one index finger-breadth anterior to SJ-20 (Jiaosun 角孙).

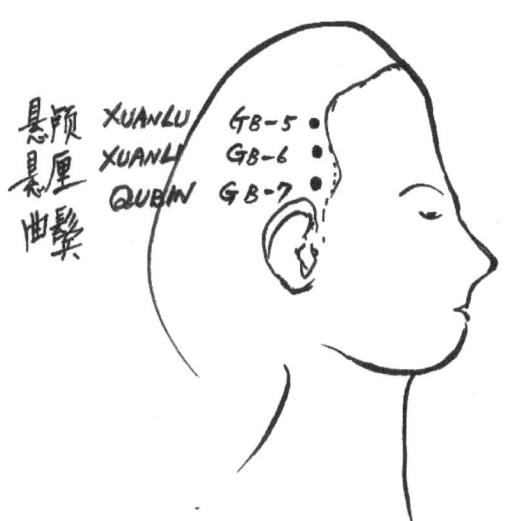

GB-8 (Shuaigu 率谷)

- On the head, 1.5 cun superior to the hairline above SJ-20 (Jiaosun 角孙).

GB-9 (Tianchong 天冲)

- Directly above the ear, in the depression 0.5 cun posterior to GB-8 (Shuaigu 率谷).

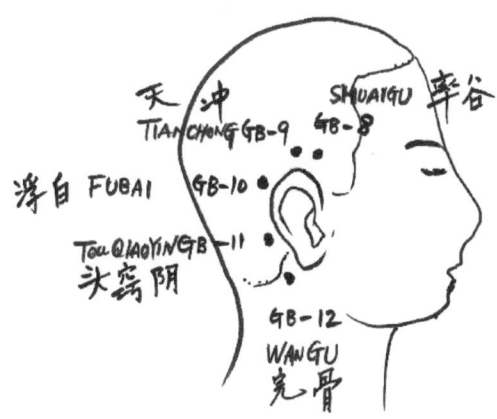

GB-10 (Fubai 浮白)

- Posterior and superior to the mastoid process, draw a curved line along the auricle from GB-9 (Tianchong 天冲) to GB-12 (Wangu 完骨), at the junction of the middle third and upper third of the curve line.

GB-11 (Touqiaoyin 头窍阴)

- Posterior and superior to the mastoid process, at the junction of middle one-third and lower one-third of the curved line connecting GB-9 (Tianchong 天冲) and GB-12 (Wangu 完骨).

GB-12 (Wangu 完骨)

- In the depression posterior and inferior to the mastoid process.

GB-13 (Benshen 本神)

- On the forehead, 0.5 cun within the anterior hairline, 3 cun lateral to DU-24 (Shenting 神庭).

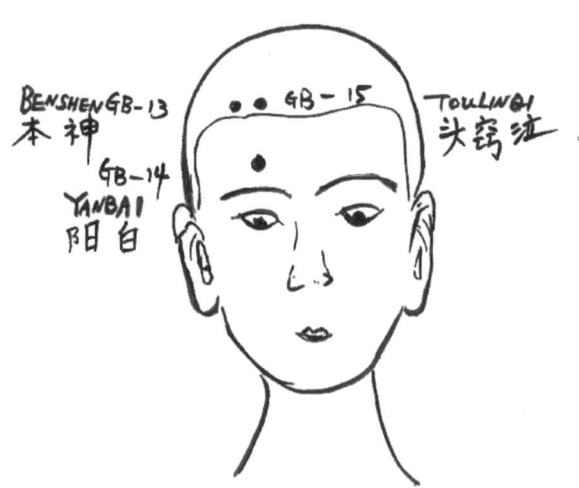

GB-14 (Yangbai 阳白)

- On the forehead, directly above the pupil, 1 cun superior to the middle of the eyebrow.

GB-15 (Toulinqi 头临泣)

- On the forehead, directly above GB-14 (Yangbai 阳白), 0.5 cun within the anterior hairline.

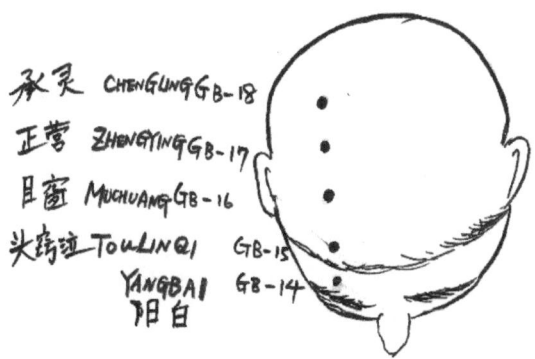

GB-16 (Muchuang 目窗)

- 1.5 cun within the anterior hairline, 2.25 cun lateral to the midline of the head.

GB-17 (Zhengying 正营)

- 2.5 cun within the anterior hairline, 2.25 cun lateral to the midline of the head.

GB-18 (Chengling 承灵)

- 4 cun within the anterior hairline, 2.25 cun lateral to the midline of the head.

GB-19 (Naokong 脑空)

- On the occipital region, 2.25 cun lateral to the midline of the head, level as DU-17 (Naohu 脑户).

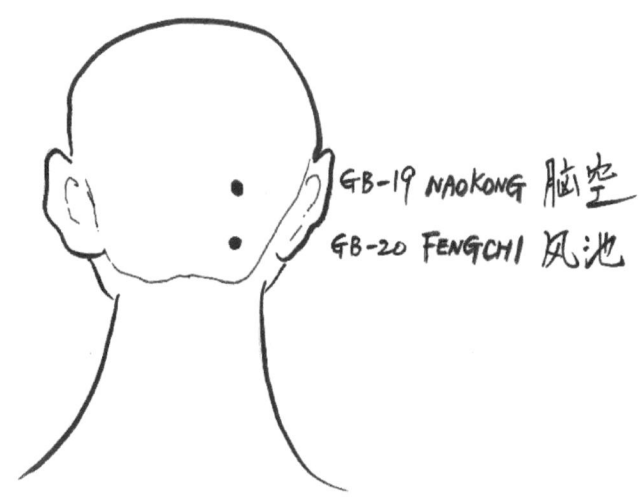

GB-20 (Fengchi 风池)

- Below the occiput, at the same level as Du-16 (Fengfu 风府), in the depression between the origins of the sternocleidomastoid and trapezius muscles.

GB-21 (Jianjing 肩井)

- On the shoulder, directly above the nipple, midway between DU-14(Dazhui 大椎) and the tip of the acromion.

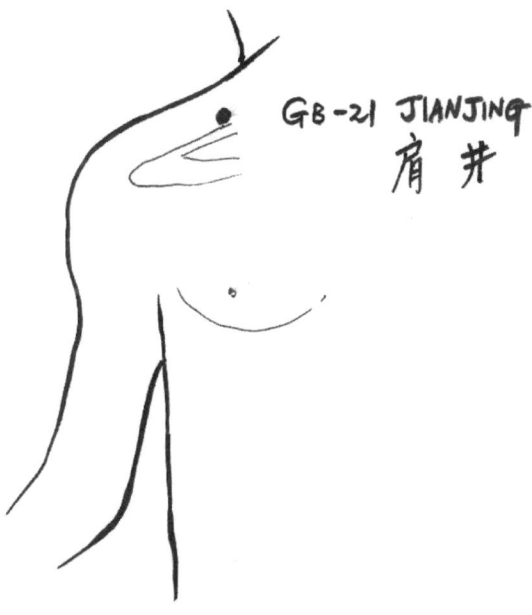

GB-21 JIANJING 肩井

GB-22 (Yuanye 渊腋)

- On the lateral side of the chest, on the axillary midline when the arm is raised, 3 cun below the axilla, at the level of the nipple, in the 4th intercostal space.

GB-23 (Zhejin 辄筋)

- 1 cun anterior to GB-22 (Yuanye 渊腋), at the level of the nipple, in the 4th intercostal space.

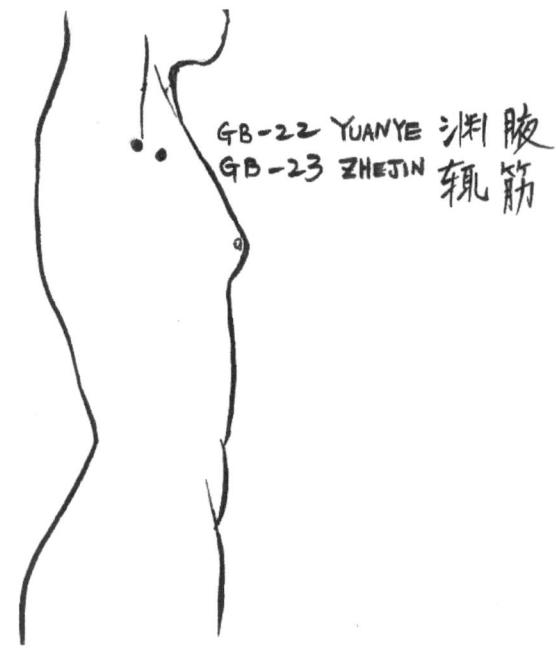

GB-24 (Riyue 日月)

- Front-Mu point of the Gall Bladder.
- Directly below the nipple, in the 7th intercostal space, 4 cun lateral to the midline.

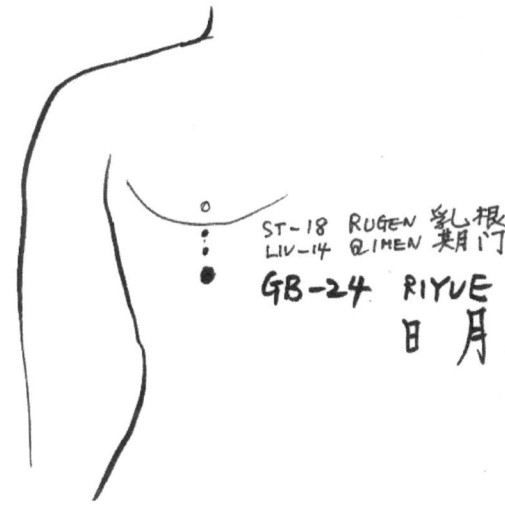

GB-25 (Jingmen 京门)

- Front-Mu point of the Kidney.
- On the lower border of the free end of the 12th rib.

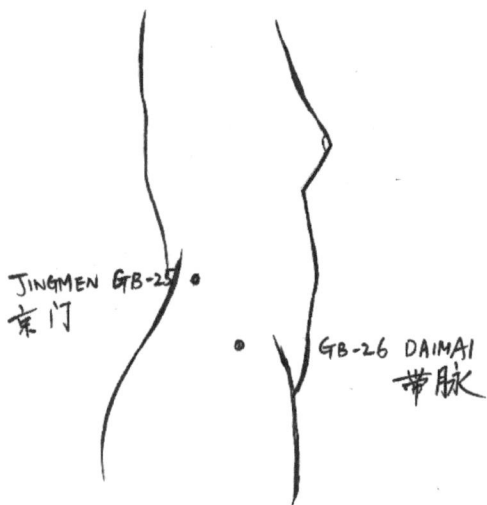

JINGMEN GB-25 京门

GB-26 DAIMAI 带脉

GB-26 (Daimai 带脉)

- On the lateral side of the abdomen, directly below LIV-13(Zhangmen 章门), at the level of the umbilicus.

GB-27 (Wushu 五俞)

- On the lateral side of the abdomen, anterior to the superior iliac spine, 3 cun below the level of the umbilicus, level with REN-4 (Guanyuan 关元).

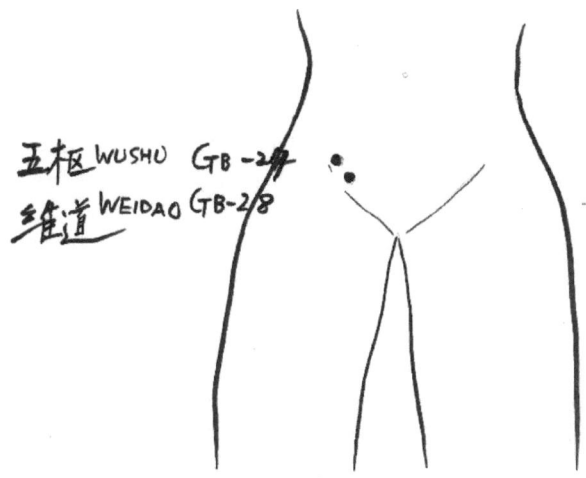

五框 WUSHU GB-27
维道 WEIDAO GB-28

GB-28 (Weidao 维道)

- On the lateral side of the abdomen, 0.5 cun anterior and inferior to GB-27 (Wushu 五俞), on the line parallel to the groin.

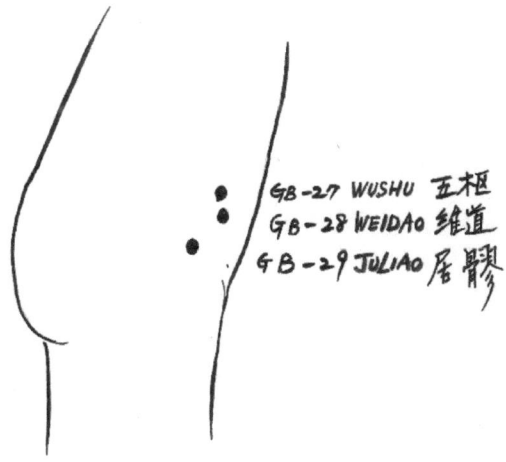

GB-27 WUSHU 五框
GB-28 WEIDAO 维道
GB-29 JULIAO 居髎

GB-29 (Juliao 居髎)

- On the hip, at the midpoint of the line connecting the anterior superior iliac spine and the prominence of the greater trochanter.

GB-30 (Huantiao 环跳)

- On the postero-lateral side of the hip joint, one third of the distance between the prominence of the great trochanter and the sacrococcygeal hiatus.

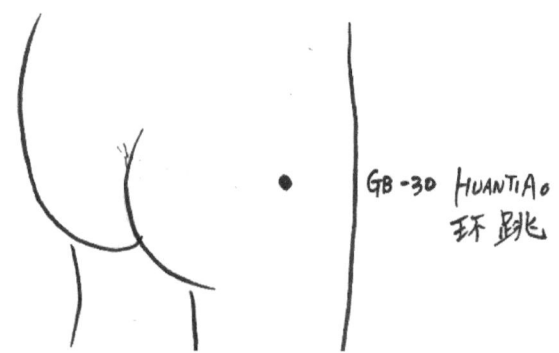

GB-30 HUANTIAO 环跳

GB-31 (Fengshi 风市)

- On the lateral midline of the thigh, 7 cun superior to the popliteal crease, when the patient stands erect with the arms hanging down freely, the point is the tip of the middle finger.

GB-32 (Zhongdu 中读)

- On the lateral side of the thigh, 2 cun inferior to GB-31 (Fengshi 风市).

GB-33 (Xiyangguan 膝阳关)

- On the lateral side of the knee, 3 cun above GB-34 (Yanglingquan 阳陵泉), at the level of the upper border of the patella, in the depression above the external epicondyle of femur.

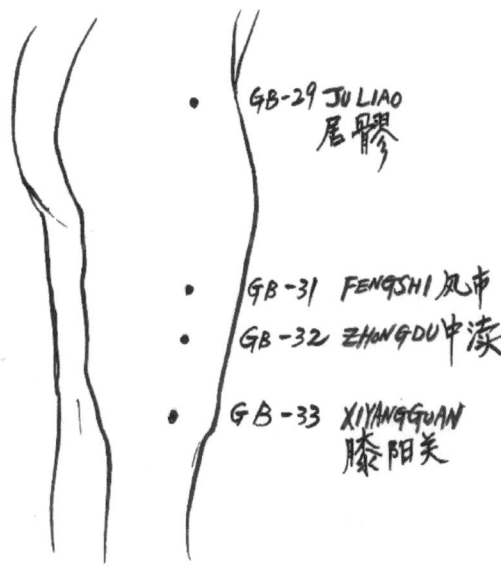

GB-34 (Yanglingquan 阳陵泉)

- He-Sea point of the Gall Bladder channel.
- On the lateral side of the lower leg, in the depression anterior and inferior to the head of the fibula.

GB-35 (Yangjiao 阳交)

- On the lateral side of the lower leg, 7 cun above to the prominence of the lateral malleolus, on the posterior border of the fibla.

GB-36 (Waiqiu 外丘)

- Xi-Cleft point of the Gall Bladder channel.
- On the lateral aspect of the lower leg, 7 cun superior to the prominence of the lateral malleolus, on the anterior border of the fibula.

GB-37 (Guangming 光明)

- Luo-connecting point of the Gall Bladder channel.
- On the lateral side of the lower leg, 5 cun superior to the prominence of the lateral malleolus, on the anterior border of the fibula.

GB-38 (Yangfu 阳辅)

- On the lateral side of the lower leg, 4 cun superior to the prominence of the lateral malleolus, on the anterior border of the fibula.

GB-39 (Xuanzhong 悬钟)

- On the lateral side of the lower leg, 3 cun superior to the prominence of the lateral malleolus, on the anterior border of the fibula.

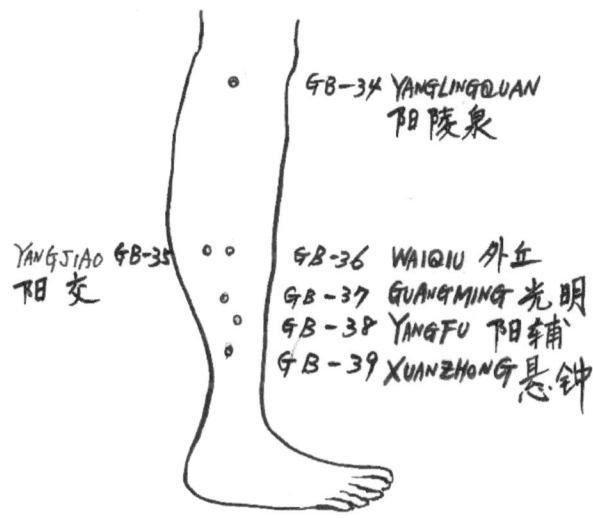

GB-40 (Qiuxu 丘墟)

- Yuan-Source point of the Gall Bladder channel.

- At the ankle joint, anterior and inferior to the lateral malleolus.

GB-41 (Zulinqi 足临泣)

- On the lateral side of the dorsum of the foot, 4th and 5th metatarsal bones, in a depression lateral to the tendon of the extensor digitiform longus of the fifth toe.

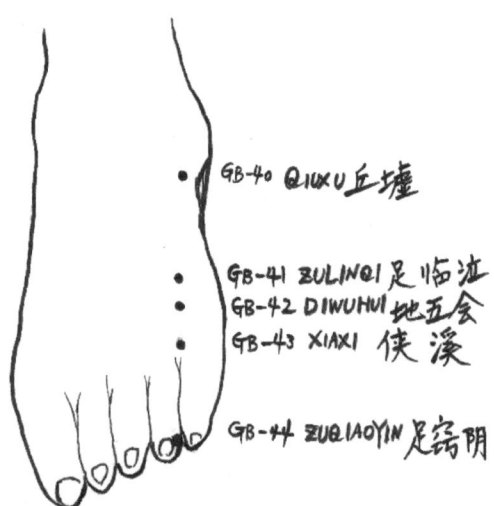

GB-42 (Diwuhui 地五会)

- Between the 4th and 5th metatarsal bones, on the medial side of the tendon of m.extensor digitorum longus.

GB-43 (Xiaxi 侠溪)

- Between the fourth and fifth toes, 0.5 cun proximal to the margin of the web.

GB-44 (Zuqiaoyin 足窍阴)

- On the lateral side of the fourth toe, 0.1 cun from the corner of the nail.

XII. The Liver Channel of Foot-Jueyin
足厥阴肝经经穴

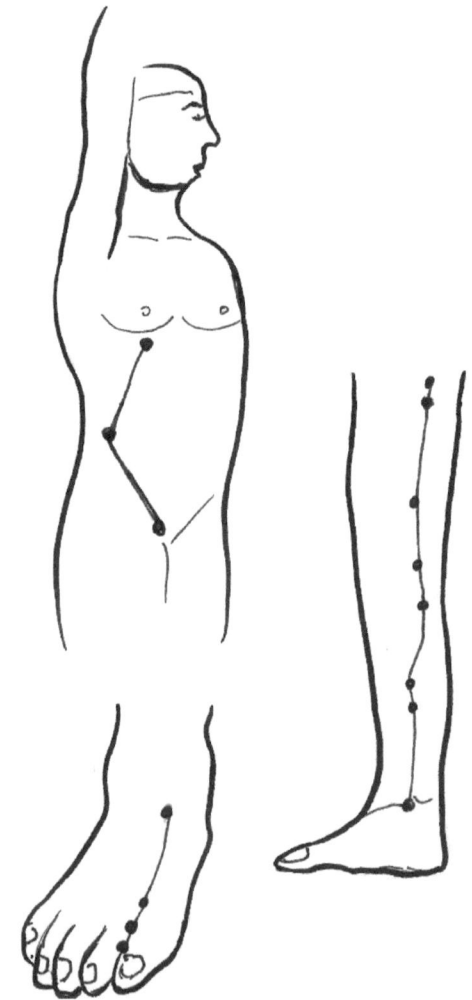

Originates from the dorsal region of the great toe, and then runs upward along the foot, leg to the groin and then runs upward around the stomach up to just below the nipple. It contains 14 different acupoints.

LIV-1 (Dadun 大敦)

- On the lateral side of dorsum of the the great toe, 0.1 cun beside the corner of the nail.

LIV-2 (Xingjian 行间)

- On the lateral side of dorsum of the foot, between the first and second toes, 0.5 cun proximal of the margin of the web.

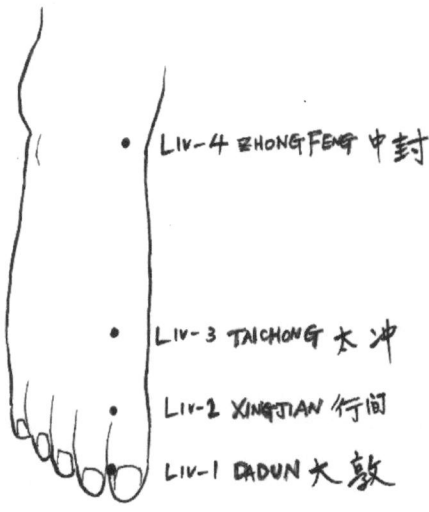

LIV-3 (Taichong 太冲)

- Yuan-Source of the Liver channel.
- On the dorsum of the foot, in the depression distal to the junction, between the first and second metatarsal bones.

LIV-4 (Zhongfeng 中封)

- On the ankle, anterior to the medial malleolus, in the depression on the medial side of the tendon of the m.tibialis anterior.

LIV-5 (Ligou 蠡沟)

- Luo-Connecting point of the Liver channel.
- 5 cun above the prominence of the medial malleolus, in the middle of the medial aspect of the tibia.

LIV-6 (Zhongdu 中都)

- Xi-Cleft point of the Liver channel.
- 7 cun above the prominence of the medial malleolus, on the midline of the medial aspect of the tibia.

LIV-7 (Xiguan 膝关)

- Posterior and inferior to the medial epicondyle of the tibia, 1 cun posterior to SP-9 (Yinlingquan 阴陵泉).

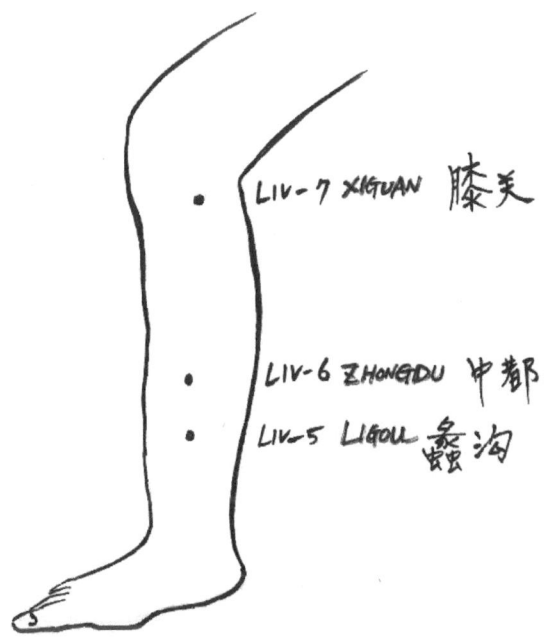

LIV-8 (Ququan 曲泉)

- He-Sea point of the Liver channel.
- When the knee is flexed, in the depression above the medial end of the transverse crease of the knee joint.

LIV-9 (Yinbao 阴包)

- On the medial side of the thigh, directly above the medial epicondyle of the femur, 4 cun above to LIV-8 (Ququan 曲泉).

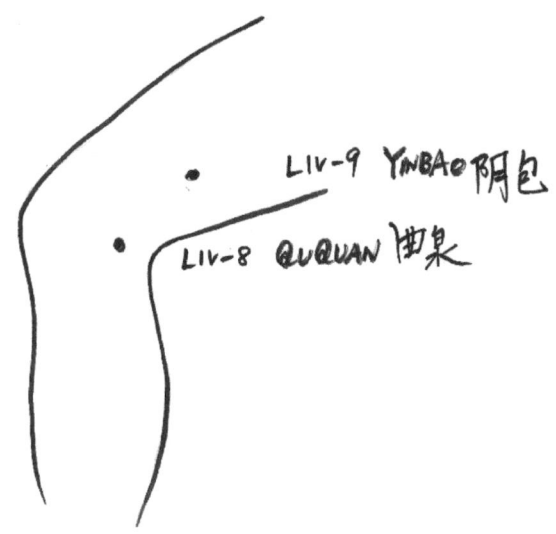

LIV-10 (Zuwuli 足五里)

- 3 cun directly below ST-30 (Qichong 气冲), at the proximal end of the thigh, below the pubic tubercle and on the lateral border of m.adductor longus.

LIV-11 (Yinlian 阴廉)

- 2 cun directly below ST-30 (Qichong 气冲), at the proximal end of the thigh, below the pubic tubercle and on the lateral border of m.adductor longus.

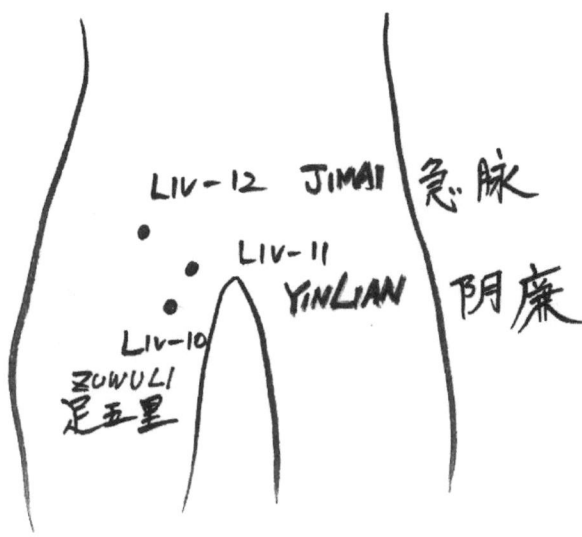

LIV-12 (Jimai 急脉)

- 2.5 cun lateral to the midway of the lower border of the pubic symphysis, 1 cun inferior to Ren-2 (Qugu 曲骨).

LIV-13 (Zhangmen 章门)

- On the lateral side of the abdomen, when the patient is flexing elbow, and touching the tip of the elbow to the hypochondriac region, the tip of the elbow.

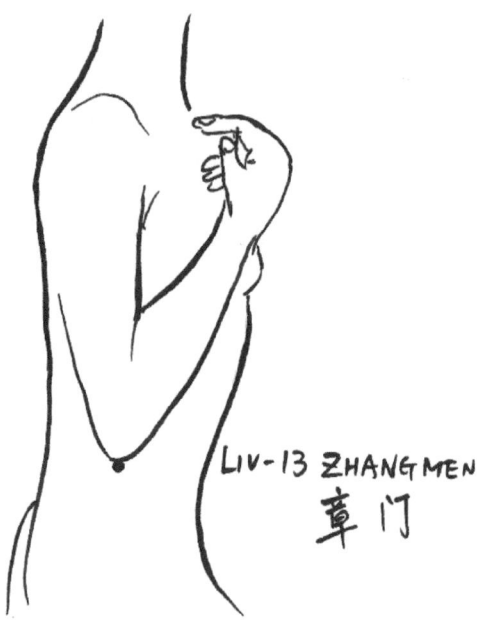

LIV-13 ZHANGMEN
章门

LIV-14 (Qimen 期门)

- Front-Mu point of the Liver.

- Directly below the nipple, in the 6th intercostal space, 4 cun lateral to the midline.

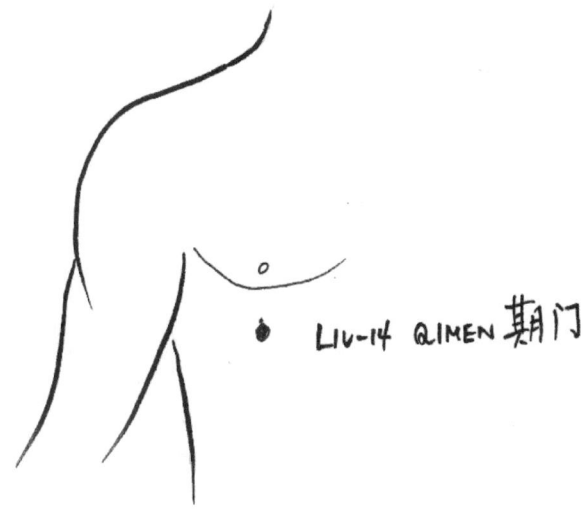

LIV-14 QIMEN 期门

XIII.   Point of the Du Channel 督脉经穴

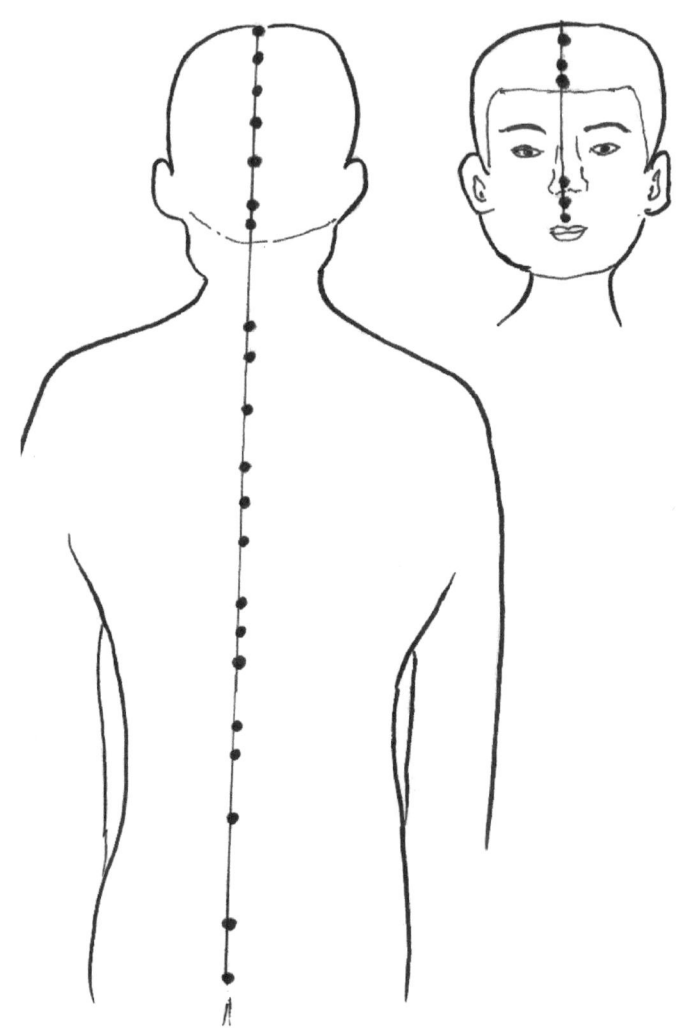

Originates from the lower abdomen and emerges from the perineum and runs straight up the spinal column to the nape, over the skull to above lip. It contains 28 different acupoints.

DU-1 (Changqiang 长强)

- Luo-Connecting point of the Governing vessel.
- At the midpoint between the tip of the coccyx and the anus.

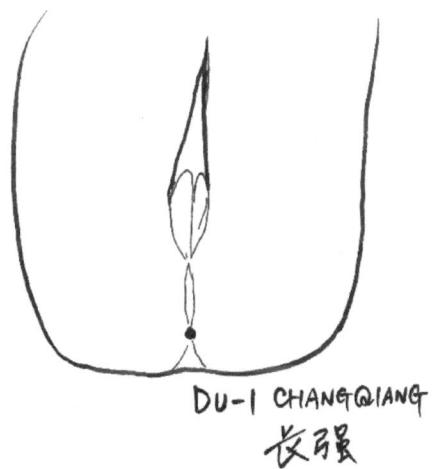

DU-1 CHANGQIANG
长强

DU-2 (Yaoshu 腰俞)

- On the sacrum, on the midline, at the sacral hiatus.

DU-3 (Yaoyangguan 腰阳关)

- On the lower back, in the depression below the spinous process of the fourth lumbar vertebra.

DU-4 (Mingmen 命门)

- On the lower back, in the depression below the spinous process of the second lumbar vertebra.

DU-5 (Xuanshu 悬俞)

- On the lower back, in the depression below the spinous process of the first lumbar vertebra.

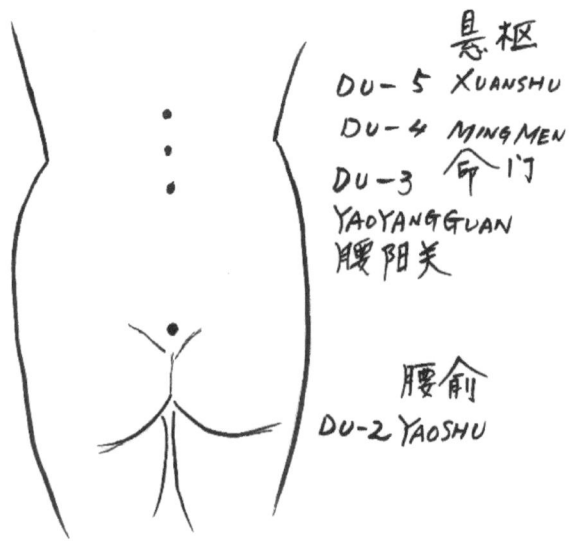

DU-6 (Jizhong 脊中)

- On the back, in the depression below the spinous process of the eleventh thoracic vertebra.

DU-7 (Zhongshu 中俞)

- On the back, in the depression below the spinous process of the tenth thoracic vertebra.

DU-8 (Jinsuo 筋缩)

- On the back, in the depression below the spinous process of the ninth thoracic vertebra.

DU-9 (Zhiyang 至阳)

- On the back, in the depression below the spinous process of the seventh thoracic vertebra.

DU10 (Lingtai 灵台)

- On the back, in the depression below the spinous process of the sixth thoracic vertebra.

DU-11 (Shendao 神道)

- On the back, in the depression below the spinous process of the fifth thoracic vertebra.

DU-12 (Shenzhu 身柱)

- On the back, in the depression below the spinous process of the third thoracic vertebra.

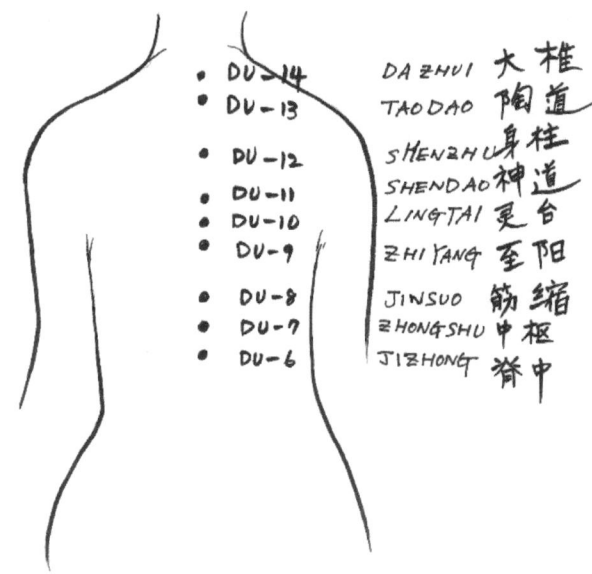

DU-13 (Taodao 陶道)

- On the back, in the depression below the spinous process of the first thoracic vertebra.

DU-14 (Dazhui 大椎)

- Point of the Sea of Qi.
- Meeting point of the Governing vessel with Six Yang channel.
- At the level of the shoulder, in the depression below the spinous process of the seventh cervical vertebra.

DU-15 (Yamen 哑门)

- On the neck, 0.5 cun above the midpoint of the posterior hairline, below the first cervical vertebra.

DU-16 (Fengfu 风府)

- Point of the Sea of Marrow.
- On the neck, 1cun above the midpoint of the posterior hairline, below the external occipital protuberance.

DU-17 (Naohu 脑户)

- On the head, 2.5 cun above the midpoint of the posterior hairline, 1.5 cun above DU-16 (Fengfu 风府), in the depression superior to the external occipital protuberance.

DU-18 (Qiangjian 强间)

- On the head, 4 cun above the midpoint of the posterior hairline, 1.5 cun above DU-17 (Naohu 脑户).

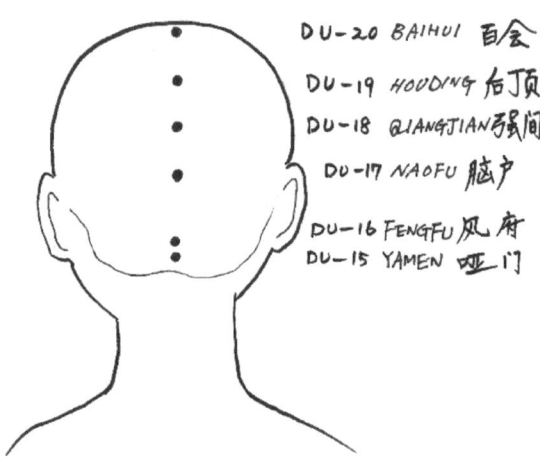

DU-19 (Houding 后顶)

- On the head, 5.5 cun above the midpoint of the posterior hairline, 1.5 cun above DU-18 (Qiangjian 强间).

DU-20 (Baihui 白会)

- Point of the Sea of Marrow.

- On the midline of the head, 5 cun above the midpoint of the anterior hairline, at the midpoint connecting the apexes of both ears.

DU-21 (Qianding 前顶)

- On the head, 3.5 cun above the midpoint of the anterior hairline, 1.5 cun anterior to DU-20 (Baihui 白会).

DU-22 (Xinhui 囟会)

- On the head, 2 cun above the midpoint of the anterior hairline, 3 cun anterior to DU-20 (Baihui 白会).

DU-23 (Shangxing 上星)

- On the head, 1 cun above the midpoint of the anterior hairline.

DU-24 (Shenting 神庭)

- At the top of the head, 0.5 cun above the midpoint of the anterior hairline.

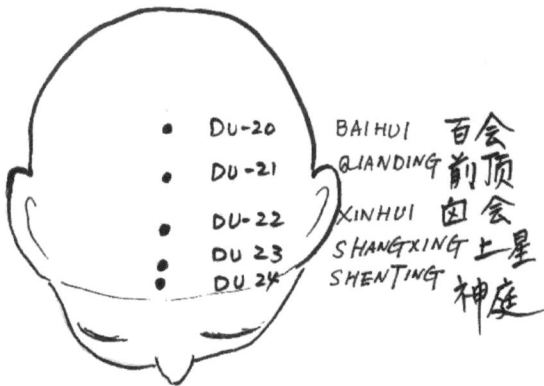

DU-25 (Suliao 素髎)

• On the face, on the tip of the nose.

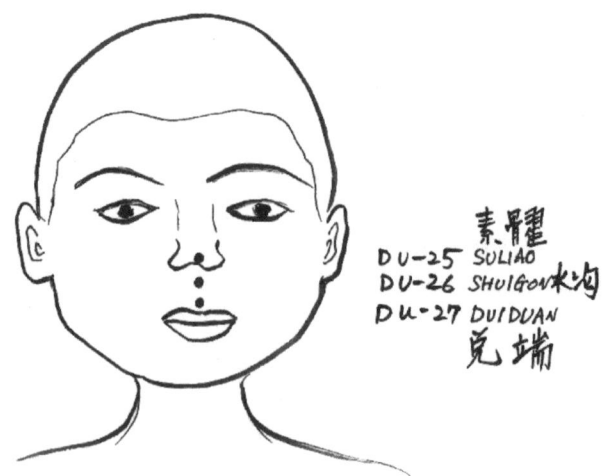

DU-26 (Shuigou 水沟)

- Above the upper lip on the midline, at the junction of the upper third and middle third of the philtrum.

DU-27 (Duiduan 兑端)

- At the junction of the lower end of the philtrum and the upper lip.

DU-28 (Yinjiao 龈交)

- Inside the upper lip, at the junction of the labial frenum and the upper gum.

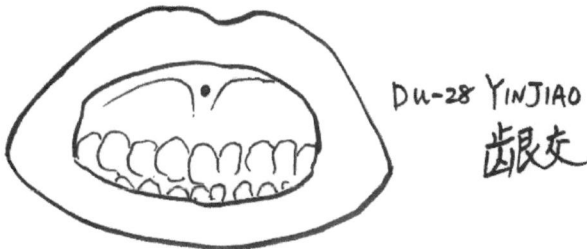

DU-28 YINJIAO

龈交

The Conception Vessel
XIV. Point of the Ren Channel 任脉经穴

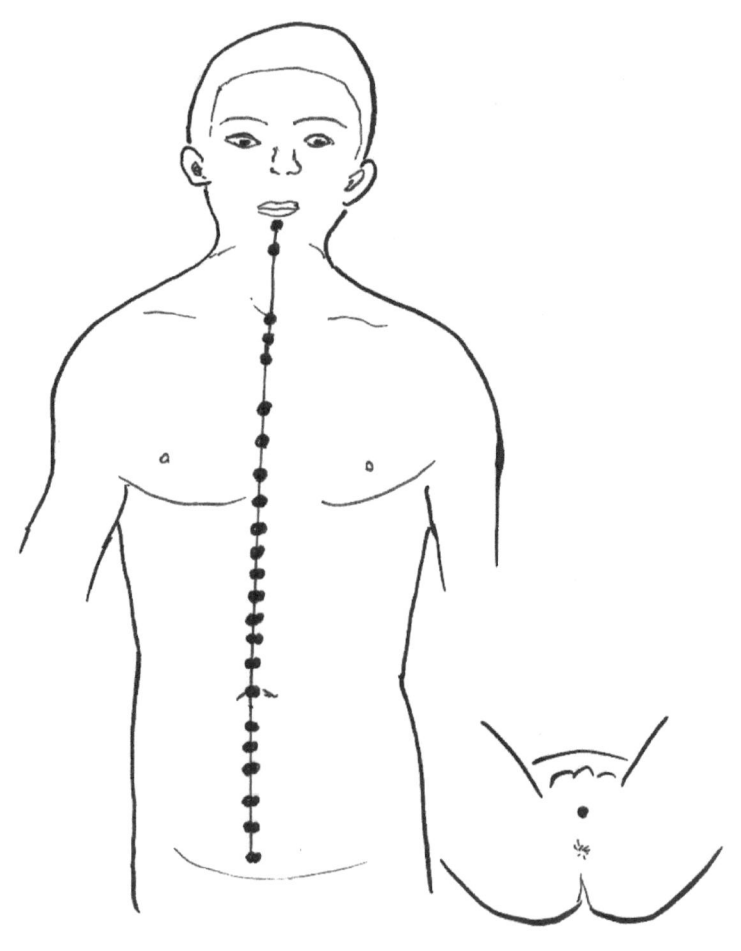

Starts above the middle of the pubic region and ascends straight up the middle of the body to below the lower lip. It contains 24 different acupoints.

REN-1 (Huiyin 会阴)

- On the perineum, between the anus and the root of the serotum in males and between the anus and posterior labial commissure in females.

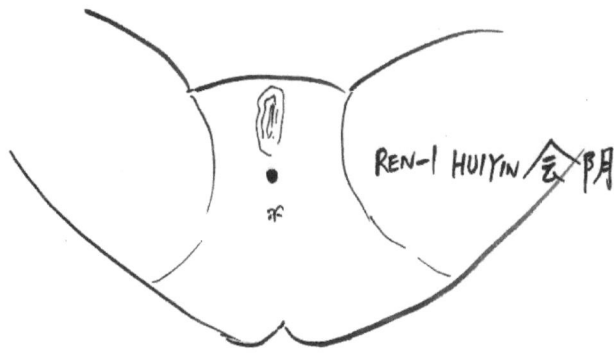

REN-2 (Qugu 曲骨)

- On the lower abdomen, on the anterior midline, at the midpoint of the upper border of the pubic symphysis.

REN-3 (Zhongji 中极)

- Front-Mu point of the Bladder.
- On the lower abdomen, 4 cun below the umbilicus.

REN-4 (Guanyuan 关元)

- Front-Mu point of the Small Intestine.
- On the lower abdomen, 3 cun below the umbilicus.

REN-5 (Shimen 石门)

- Front-Mu point of the Sanjiao.
- On the lower abdomen, 2 cun below the umbilicus.

REN-6 (Qihai 气海)

- Sea of Qi.
- On the lower abdomen, 1.5 cun below the umbilicus.

REN-7 (Yinjiao 阴交)

- On the lower abdomen, 1 cun below the umbilicus.

REN-8 (Shenque 神阙)

- In the centre of the umbilicus.

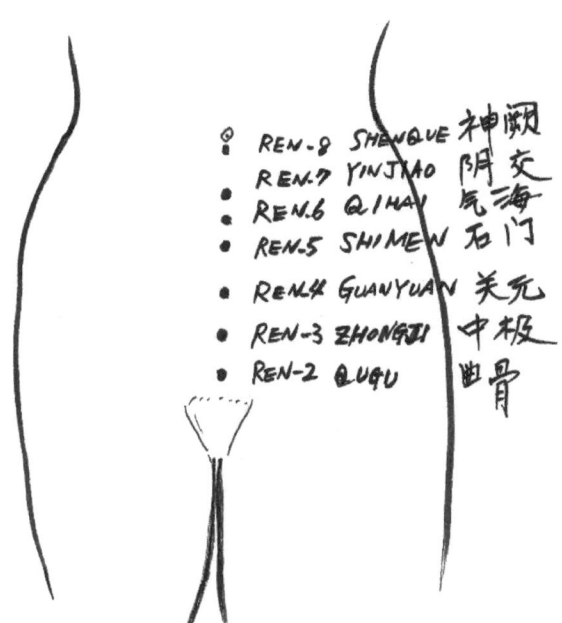

REN-8 SHENQUE 神阙
REN-7 YINJIAO 阴交
REN-6 QIHAI 气海
REN-5 SHIMEN 石门
REN-4 GUANYUAN 关元
REN-3 ZHONGJI 中极
REN-2 QUQU 曲骨

REN-9 (Shuifen 水分)

- In the upper abdomen, 1 cun above the umbilicus.

REN-10 (Xiawan 下脘)

- On the upper abdomen, 2 cun above the umbilicus.

REN-11 (Jianli 建里)

- On the upper abdomen, 3 cun above the umbilicus.

REN-12 (Zhongwan 中脘)

- Front-Mu point of the Stomach.
- On the upper abdomen, 4 cun above the umbilicus.

REN-13 (Shangwan 上脘)

- On the upper abdomen, 5 cun above the umbilicus.

REN-14 (Juqueju 巨阙)

- Front-Mu point of the Heart.
- On the upper abdomen, 6 cun above the umbilicus.

REN-15 (Jiuwei 鸠尾)

- Luo-Connecting point of the Conception vessel.
- On the upper abdomen, 7 cun above the umbilicus, 1 cun below the sternocostal angle.

REN-16 (Zhongting 中庭)

- On the chest, on the middle of the sternocostal angle.

REN-17(Shanzhong 膻中)

- Front-Mu point of the Pericardium.
- At the level of the fourth intercostal space, the midpoint of the line connecting both nipples.

REN-18 (Yutang 玉堂)

- On the midline of the chest, at the level of the third intercostal space.

REN-19 (Zigong 紫宫)

- On the midline of the chest, at the level of the second intercostal space.

REN-20 (Huagai 华盖)

- On the midline of the chest, at the level of the first intercostal space.

REN-21 (Xuanji 璇玑)

- On the chest, in the centre of the sternal manubrium, 1 cun posterior to REN-22 (Tiantu 天突).

REN-22 (Tiantu 天突)

- On the neck, in the centre of the suprasternal fossa.

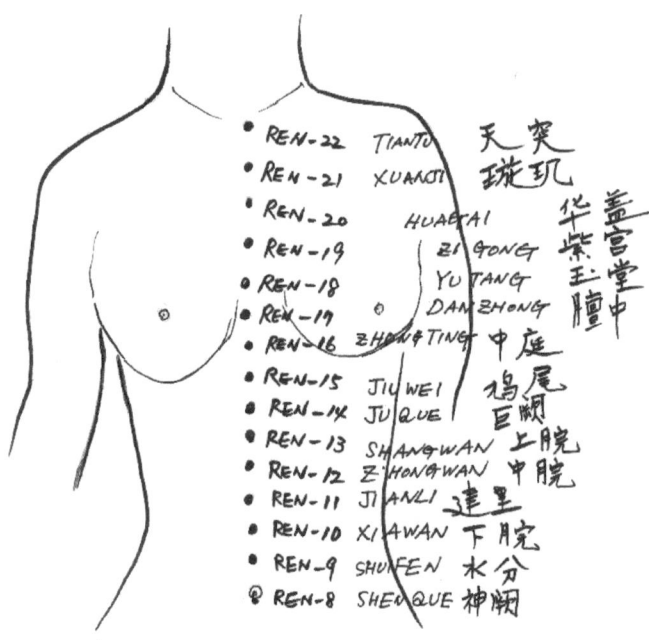

REN-23 (Lianquan 廉泉)

- On the neck, on the anterior midline, in the depression above the hyoid bone.

REN-24 (Chengjiang 承浆)

- On the face, in the depression at the midpoint of the mentolabial groove.

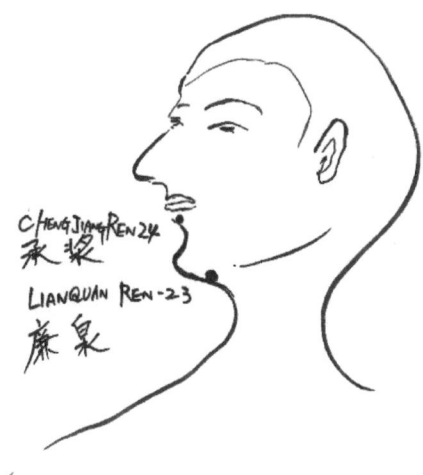

Section 4 Location of the Extra-ordinary Point 常用经外奇穴定位

(1). Points of the Head and Neck 头颈部穴
EX-HN1 Sishencong 四神聪

- Four points on the head 1 cun respectively, anterior and lateral to DU-20 (Baihui 白会).

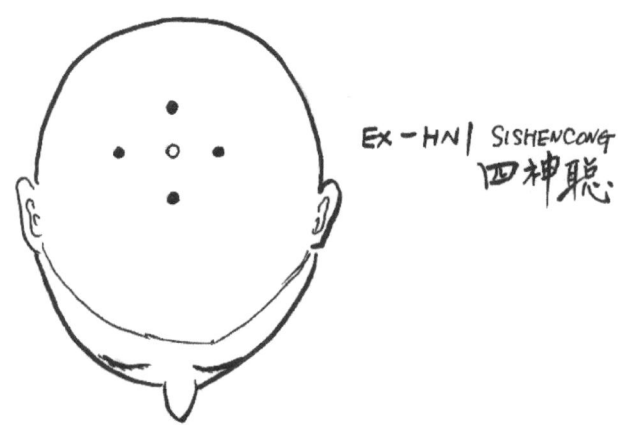

EX-HN2 Dangyang 当阳

- At the front part of the head, directly above the pupil, 0.5 cun above GB-15 (Toulinqi 头临泣).

EX-HN3 Yintang 印堂

- On the forehead, at the midpoint between the two eyebrows.

EX-HN4 Yuyao 鱼腰

- On the forehead, directly above the pupil, in the centre of the eyebrow.

EX-HN5 Taiyang 太阳

- At the temporal part of the head, in the depression 1 cun posterior to the midpoint between the lateral end of the eyebrow and the outer canthus of the eye.

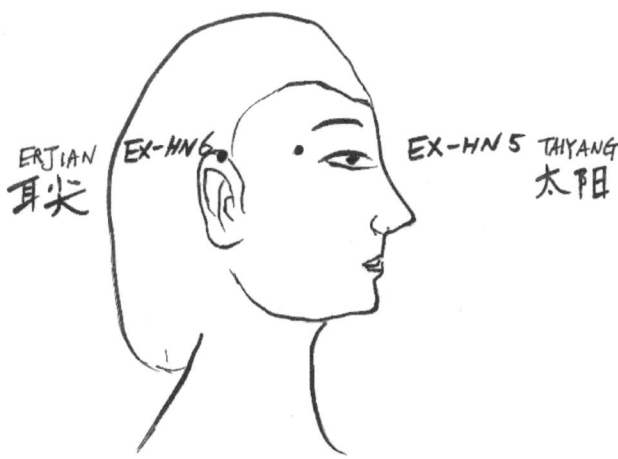

EX-HN6 Erjian 耳尖

- When the ear is folded forward, the point is located at the apex of the ear.

EX-HN7 Qiuhou 球后

- On the face, at the junction of the lateral fourth and medial three fourths of the infraorbital margin.

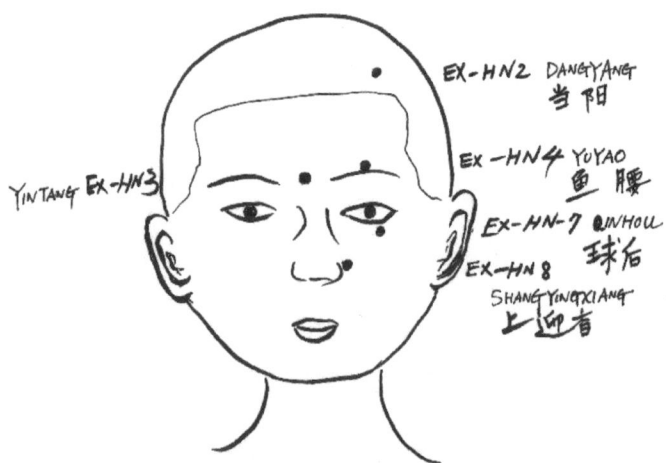

EX-HN8 Shangyingxiang 上迎香

- On the face, at the upper end of the nasolabial groove.

EX-HN9 Neiyingxiang 内迎香

- In the nostril, at the junction between the alar cartilage of the nose and the nose concha.

EX-HN10 Juquan 聚泉

- In the mouth, at the midpoint of the midline on the tongue surface.

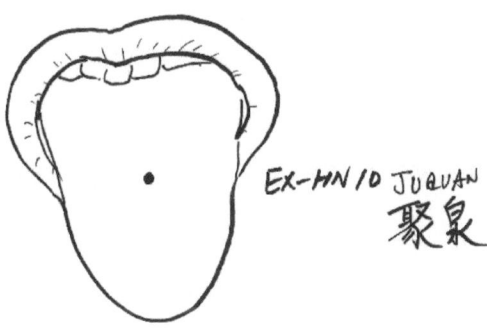

EX-HN11 Haiquan 海泉

- At the midpoint of the frenulum of the tongue, between EX-HN12 Jinjin and EX-HN13 Yuye.

EX-HN12 Jinjin 金津

- In the mouth, on the vein of the left side of the frenulum of the tongue.

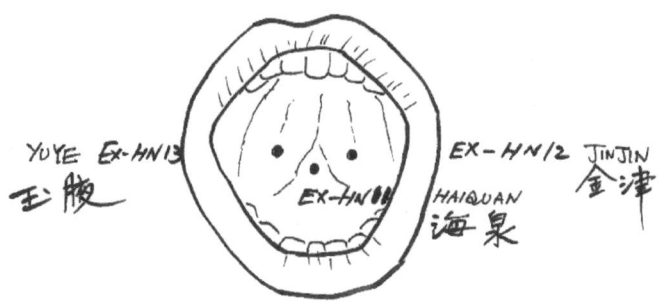

EX-HN13 Yuye 玉腋

- In the mouth, on the vein of the right side of the frenulum of the tongue.

EX-HN14 Yiming 翳明

- 1 cun posterior to SJ-17 (Yifeng 翳风).

EX-HN15 Jingbailao 颈百劳

- 2 cun above DU-14 (Dazhui 大椎), 1 cun lateral to the midline.

EX-HN16 Anmian 安眠

- Behind the ear, between GB-20 (Fengchi 风池) and SJ-17 (Yifeng 翳风).

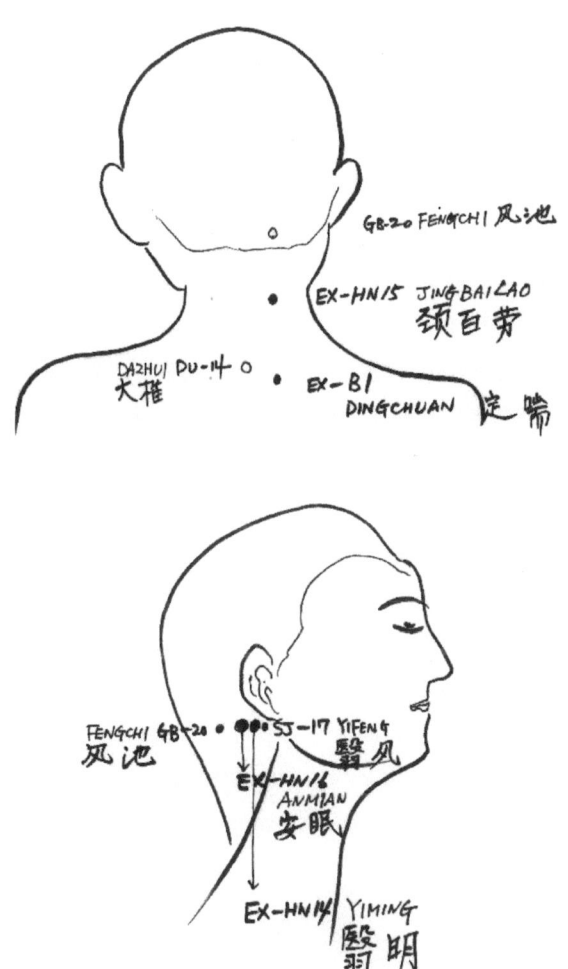

(2) Points of the Chest and Abdomen
胸腹部穴
EX-CA1 Zigong 子宫

- On the lower abdomen, 3 cun lateral to REN-3 (Zhongji 中极).

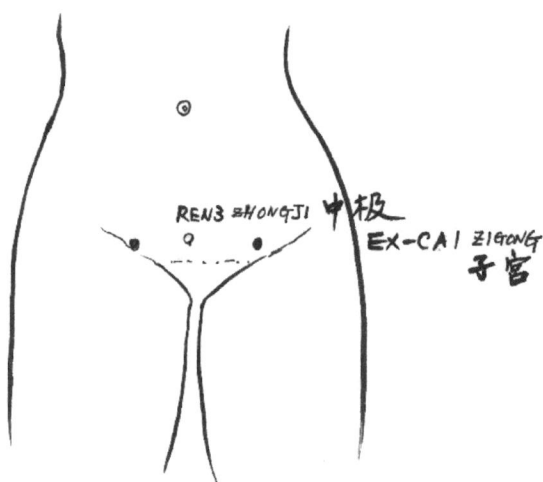

(3) Points of the Back 背部穴
EX-B1 Dingchuan 定喘

- On the back, 0.5 cun lateral to DU-14 (Dazhui 大椎).

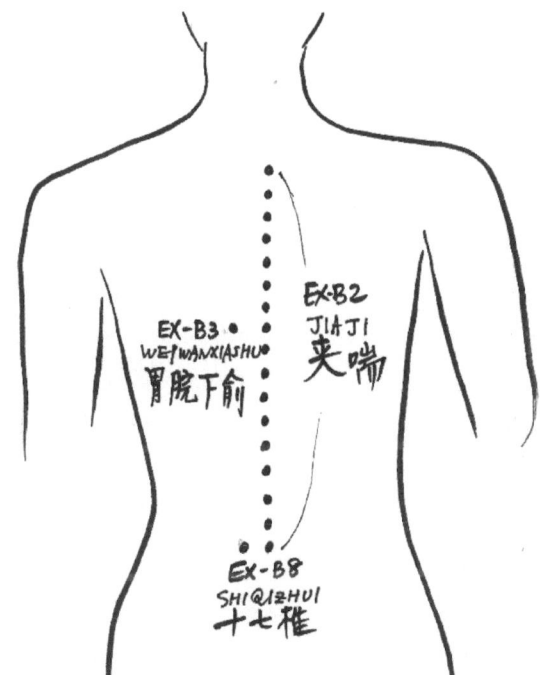

EX-B2 Jiaji 夹脊

- On each side of the back, 0.5 cun lateral to the lower border of each spinous process from the first thoracic vertebra to the fifth lumbar vertebra, totaling 17 points on each side.

EX-B3 Weiwanxiashu 胃脘下俞

- On the back, below the spinous process of the eighth thoracic vertebra, 1.5 cun lateral to the posterior midline.

EX-B4 Pigen 痞根

- On the lower back, below the spinous process of the first lumbar vertebra, 3.5 cun lateral to the posterior midline.

EX-B5 Xiajishu 下极俞

- On the midline of the lower back, below the spinous process of the third lumber vertebra.

EX-B6 Yaoyi 腰宜

- On the lower back, below the spinous process of the fourth lumbar vertebra, 3 cun lateral to the posterior midline.

EX-B7 Yaoyan 腰眼

- On the lower back, below the spinous process of the fourth lumbar vertebra, 3.5 cun lateral to the posterior midline.

EX-B8 Shiqizhui 十七椎

- On the lower back, the posterior midline below the spinous process of the fifth lumbar vertebra.

EX-B9 Yaoqi 腰奇

- On the lower back, 2 cun directly above the tip of the coccyx, in the depression between the sacral horns.

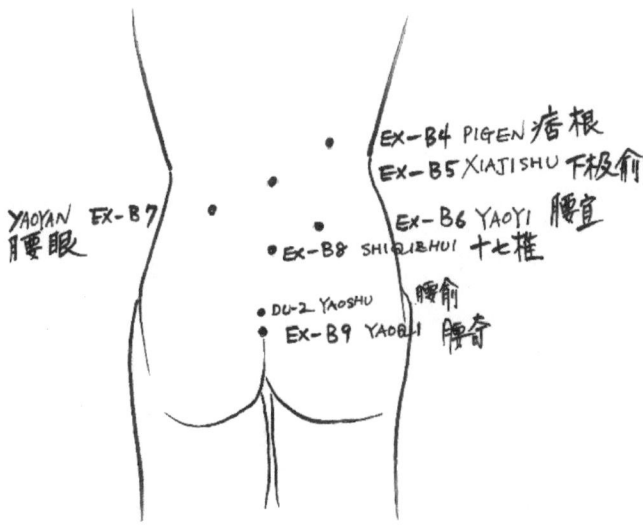

(4) Points on the Upper Extremities 上肢穴

EX-UE1 Zhoujian 肘尖

- On the posterior side of the elbow, at the tip of the ulnar olecranon when the elbow is flexed.

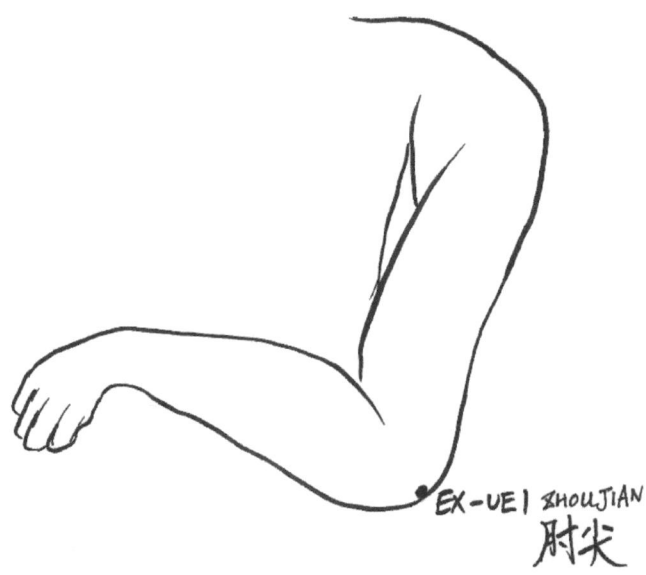

EX-UE1 ZHOUJIAN 肘尖

EX-UE2 Erbai 二白

- On the palmer side of forearm, a pair of points, 4 cun above the transverse crease of the wrist, on both sides of the tendon of m. flexor carpi radialis, two points on the hand.

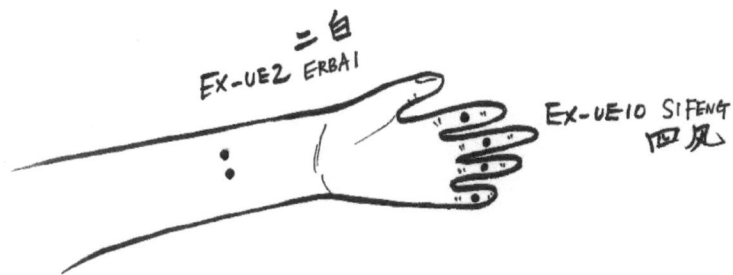

EX-UE3 Zhongquan 中泉

- On the dorsal crease of the wrist, in the depression on the radial side of the tendon of the m. extensor digitorum communis.

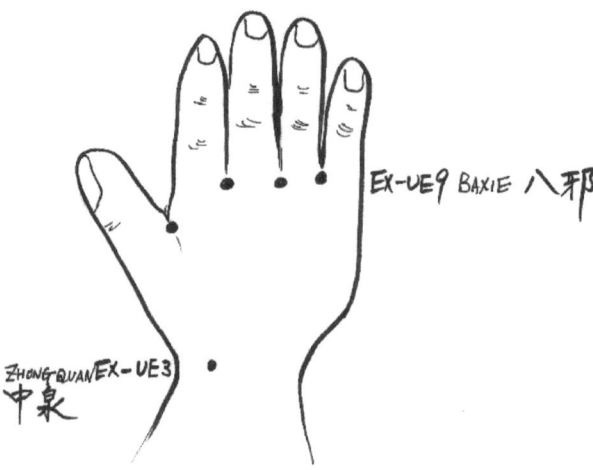

EX-UE9 BAXIE 八邪

ZHONG QUAN EX-UE3 中泉

EX-UE4 Zhongkui 中魁

- On the dorsal side of the middle finger, at the center of the proximal interphalangeal joint.

EX-UE5 Dagukong 大骨空

- On the dorsal side of the thumb, at the center of the interphalangeal joint.

EX-UE6 Xiaogukong 小骨空

- On the dorsal side of the little finger, at the midpoint of the proximal interphalangeal joint.

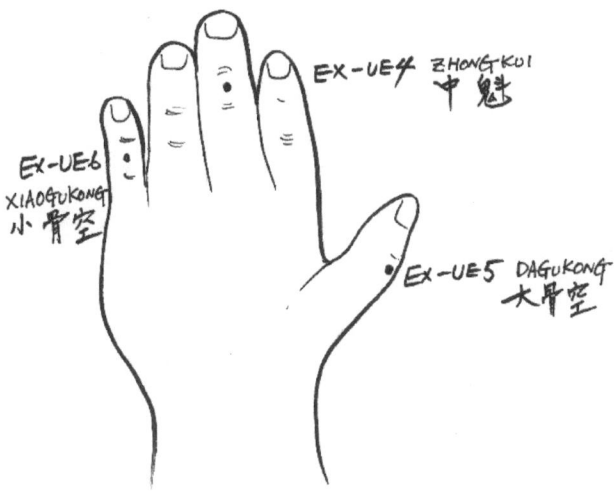

EX-UE7 Yaotongdian 腰痛点

- On the dorsum of the hand, midway between the transverse crease of the wrist and the metacarpophalangeal joint, between the second and third metacarpal bones, between the fourth and fifth metacarpal bones, two points on each hand.

EX-UE8 Wailaogong 外劳宫

- On the dorsum of the hand, between second and third metacarpal bones.

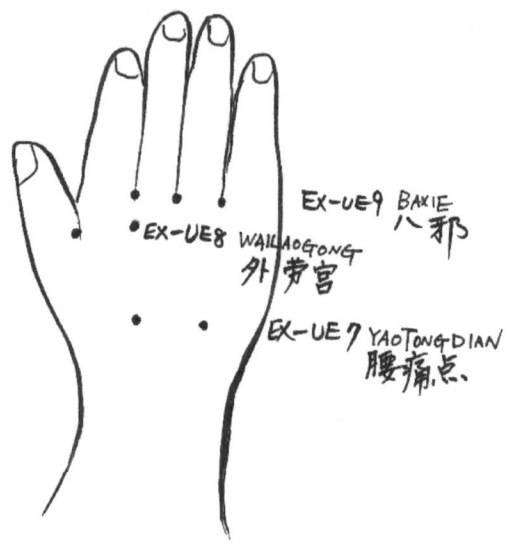

EX-UE9 BAXIE 八邪

EX-UE8 WAILAOGONG 外劳宫

EX-UE7 YAOTONGDIAN 腰痛点.

EX-UE9 Baxie 八邪

- When the hand is made into a fist, the points are located at the ends of the vertical skin crease of the webs between every two fingers.

EX-UE10 Sifeng 四缝

- On the palmar side of the hand, in the midpoint of the transverse crease of the proximal interphalangeal joint of the index, middle, ring and small fingers.

EX-UE11 Shixuan 十宣

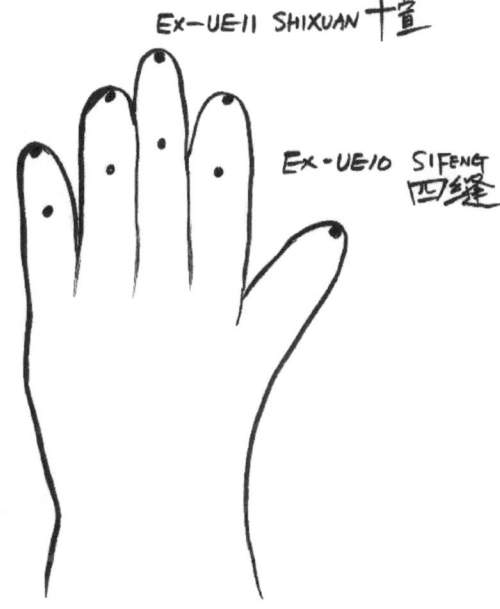

- On the tips of the ten fingers, 0.1cun distal to the nails.

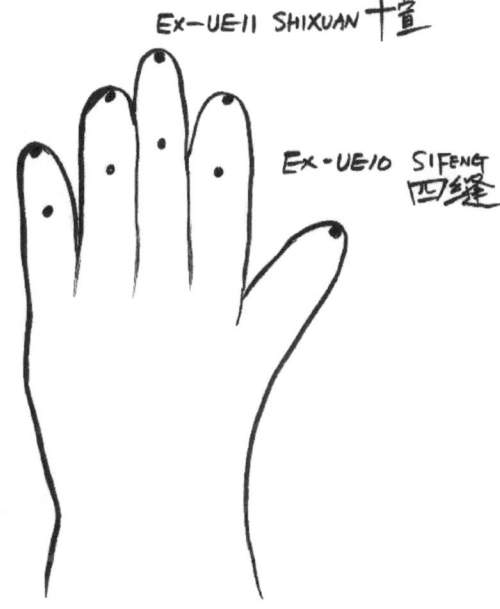

EX–UE-11 SHIXUAN 十宣

EX-UE-10 SIFENG 四缝

(5) Points on the Lower Extremities 下肢穴

EX-LE1 Kuangu 髋骨

- On the lower part of the anterior thigh, 1.5 cun lateral to ST-34 (Liang 梁丘), two points on each thigh.

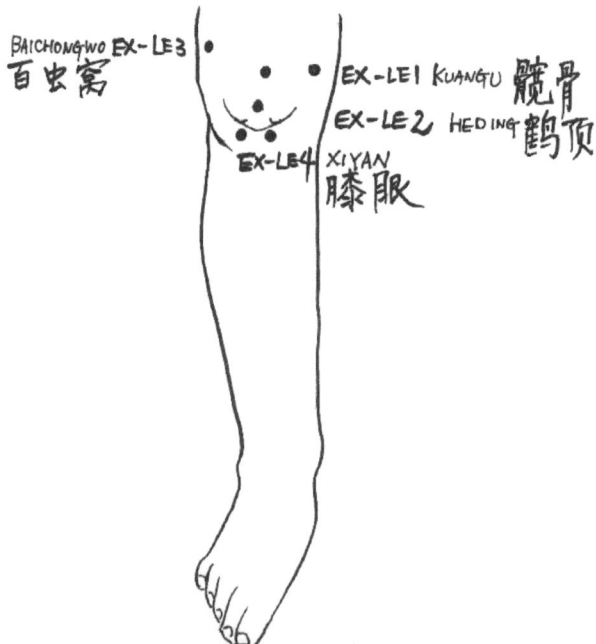

EX-LE2 Heding 鹤顶

- Above the knee, in the depression of the midpoint of the upper border of the patella.

EX-LE3 Baichongwo 百虫窝

- 3 cun above the superior border of the patella, 1 cun above SP-10 (Xuehai 血海).

EX-LE4 Xiyan 膝眼

- When the knee is flexed, in the depression medial and lateral side of the patellar ligament, the medial side is called Neixiyan 内膝眼, on the lateral side is called Waixiyan 外膝眼.

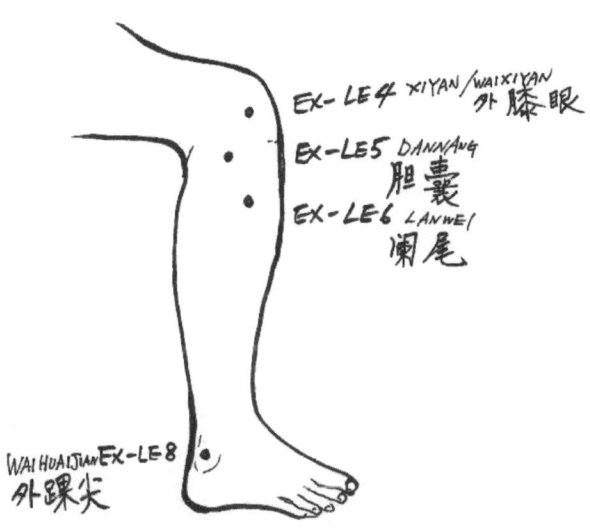

EX-LE5 Dannang 胆囊

- At the upper part of the lateral of the leg, 2 cun below GB-34 (Yanglingquan 阳陵泉).

EX-LE6 Lanwei 阑尾

- At the upper part of the anterior of the leg, 2cun below ST-36 (Zusanli 足三里).

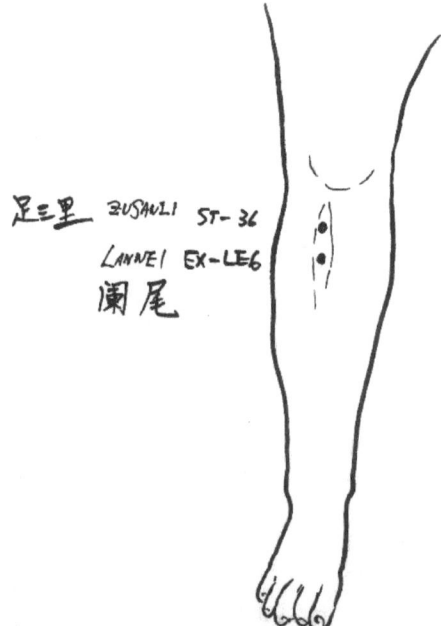

EX-LE7 Neihuaijian 内踝尖

- On the medial side of the foot, at the prominence of the medial malleolus.

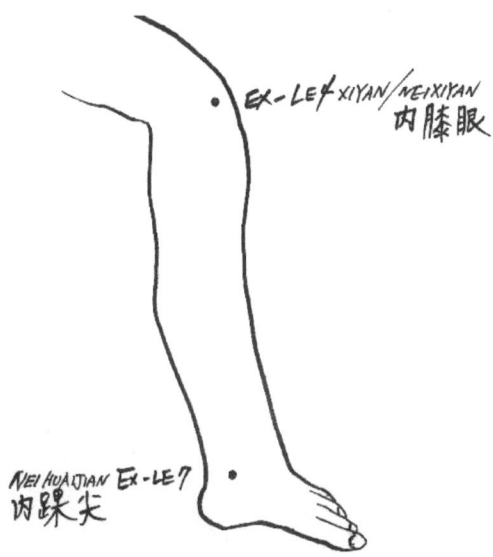

EX-LE8 Waihuaijian 外踝尖

- On the lateral side of the foot, at the prominence of the lateral malleolus.

EX-LE9 Bafeng 八风

- On the dorsum of the foot, at the margin of the webs between each two toes, four points on each foot, eight points in all.

EX-LE10 Duyin 独阴

- On the plantar side of the second toe, at the midpoint of the transverse crease.

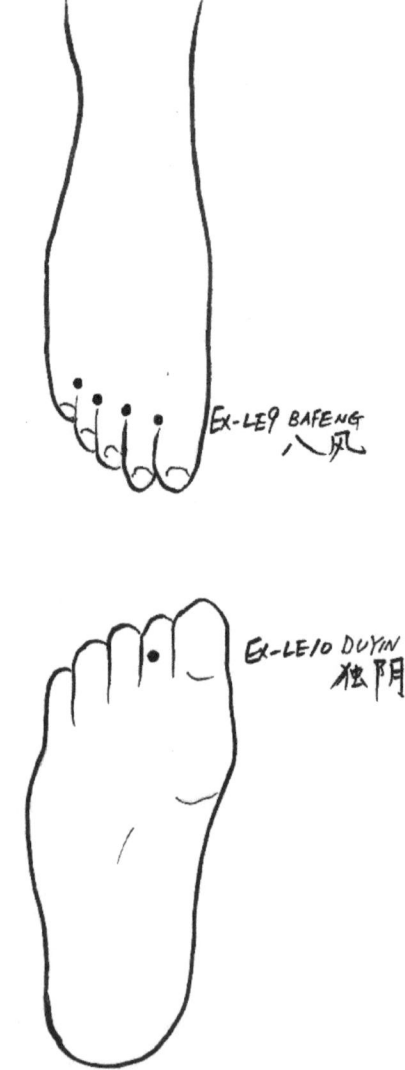

EX-LE9 BAFENG 八风

EX-LE10 DUYIN 独阴

EX-LE11 Qiduan 气端

- On the tip of the ten toes, 0.1 cun distal to the nails, ten points in all.

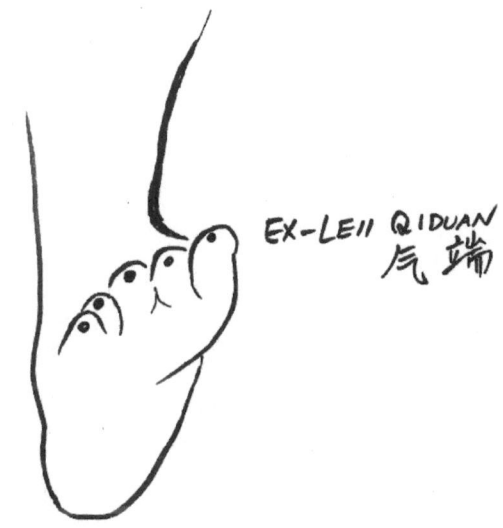